Contents

Fitness

B 50

Fitness

HEALTH FACTS

Nora J. Krantzler, PhD, MPH

and

Kathleen R. Miner, PhD, MPH, CHES

ETR ASSOCIATES

Santa Cruz, California

1994

ETR Associates (Education, Training and Research) is a nonprofit organization committed to fostering the health, well-being and cultural diversity of individuals, families, schools and communities. The publishing program of ETR Associates provides books and materials that empower young people and adults with the skills to make positive health choices. We invite health professionals to learn more about our high-quality publishing, training and research programs by contacting us at P.O. Box 1830, Santa Cruz, CA 95061-1830, 1-800-321-4407.

Published by ETR Associates, P.O. Box 1830,
Santa Cruz, California 95061-1830

Printed in the United States of America
Designed by Ann Smiley
10 9 8 7 6 5
Title No. H300

Library of Congress Cataloging-in-Publication Data

Krantzler, Nora.
Fitness : health facts / Nora J. Krantzler and Kathleen R. Miner.
p. cm.
Includes bibliographical references and index.
ISBN 1-56071-180-9
1. Physical fitness. I. Miner, Kathleen Rae, 1946–
II. Title.
RA781.K72 1994 93-46061
613.7—dc20

Editor's Preface

Everyone agrees that children and youth need to learn skills for establishing good health habits. Most people also agree that the earlier health education starts, the better its success.

The books in the *Health Facts* series were written to provide the background information educators need as they teach young people about health. The information is provided in a way that makes it easy for educators to familiarize themselves quickly with the most important facts about a health topic.

Rather than providing indepth information in each content area, the books offer guidance to the balance of emphasis. They help educators approach health topics with confidence and focus health content as they teach.

Titles in the Series

Each volume in the series contains information about a different content area. The following books comprise the series:

- *Abstinence*
- *Disease*
- *Drugs*
- *Environmental and Community Health*
- *Fitness*
- *HIV*
- *Injury Prevention*
- *Nutrition and Body Image*
- *Self-Esteem and Mental Health*
- *Sexuality*
- *STD*
- *Tobacco*
- *Violence*

Contributors

These books were written by the following talented and knowledgeable professionals in collaboration with ETR Associates' staff.

Nora Krantzler, PhD, MPH, is a freelance writer and researcher who specializes in issues related to health. She has a doctorate in medical anthropology and a master's in epidemiology. Her work has been presented in professional journals, at meetings of professional societies, in government reports and policy manuals, and in other books. Topics have included nutrition issues, child abuse and neglect, and medical practice.

Kathleen R. Miner, PhD, MPH, CHES, is associate professor and coordinator of health promotion and education in the Division of Behavioral Science and Health Education at Emory University School of Public Health. She has traveled internationally as a health educator and is the author of many articles about education and health. A former high school health and biology teacher, she has been a key contributor in designing these books to be useful to teachers.

Lucas Stang has a background in biology and health, with graduate work in science communication. He has been writing health materials for ten years. He recently served as wellness coordinator for the International School in Manila, Philippines, where he developed a kindergarten through grade 12 health curriculum and taught high school health. He has also taught human sexuality at the junior college level.

Netha L. Thacker is project editor for the *Health Facts* series. She has been involved in the development of health education materials for more than five years, on topics including puberty, adolescent sexuality, and prevention of HIV and other sexually transmitted disease. She has an extensive background in journalism, writing and editing and has been the editor of statewide newsletters for both the California AIDS Clearinghouse and the Tobacco Education Clearinghouse of California.

Acknowledgments

We would like to thank the following people, who provided reviews and content expertise.

John T. Boothby, PhD, is an associate professor at San Jose State University in San Jose, California, where he teaches microbiology and immunology.

Rama Khalsa, PhD, is a clinical psychologist and the director of the Santa Cruz County Department of Mental Health in Santa Cruz, California.

Wendy J. Schiff, MS, is a technical writing specialist in health and nutrition and teaches health at St. Louis Community College in St. Louis, Missouri.

We would also like to thank Mary Nelson, publisher of ETR Associates, for the concept idea, Kathleen Middleton, editor-in-chief of ETR Associates, for her review and conceptualization, and Susan Bagby and Jill Schettler for their help in editing.

Introduction

Looked at in terms of evolution, it is not surprising that exercise should have a positive effect on health. Throughout 99 percent of our evolution, human beings have had to be quite active.... Paleolithic men and women had a lifelong exercise program.... Such exercise didn't require any planning, it was simply a required part of hunting and gathering...an integral part of people's lives.

—Mark and Nancy Samuels

Modern men and women have adapted comfortably to a lifestyle full of energy-saving gadgets. They do not need to plant and harvest food, construct shelter, or chop and stack wood. Now people provide for their basic needs by pushing grocery carts, hiring contractors and turning up thermostats. The contemporary lifestyle does not require physical fitness, strength or endurance for subsistence, safety or success. Many people find it very easy to avoid physical effort altogether.

Physical fitness provided our ancestors with a great deal of benefit beyond maintaining the essentials for survival. This benefit was not well understood until the latter half of the twentieth century.

Recent studies have shown that physical fitness promotes lower blood pressure, lower cholesterol levels, insulin utilization and a general sense of well-being. Conversely, studies have demonstrated a relationship between sedentary lifestyles and increased incidence of heart disease, arthritis, osteoporosis, obesity, diabetes and depression.

Unlike our prehistoric ancestors, whose fitness emanated from the necessities of daily living, people today need to make a conscious effort to schedule time for exercise and other forms of physical activity. Arranging time for exercise does not need to be a huge task, nor does exercise need to be excessive to have health benefits.

People will derive some health benefits from the physical activity associated with walking instead of driving, climbing stairs instead of using elevators and raking leaves instead of using blowers. They can select recreational activities that require some level of physical exertion rather than watching television or playing cards.

In addition to the health benefits, exercise enhances mental health. People who are physically fit are better able to handle stressful situations than people who are sedentary. They are able to cope with anxiety, focus their attention and resolve their worries with less conflict than people who do not exercise. Regular exercise may be one of the pathways through which the mind and body converge.

Advances in technology will continue to relieve people of the mundane tasks of living. While these advances occur, the value of exercise and physical fitness must be remembered. Progress is wonderful, but to promote health and prevent disease, people still need to hang on to some of the behaviors of their distant ancestors.

Fitness: Health Facts provides teachers with the basics of exercise and exercise programs. The book outlines the health and physiological benefits of exercise, discusses the prevalent measures of physical fitness and suggests activities that promote physical endurance, flexibility and strength. It also presents information about the relationship between fitness and nutrition.

The Role of Education

The research conducted during the past thirty years has offered greater insight into the causes of chronic disease, injury and violence. This research indicates that these conditions are primarily caused by human behavior. What people do or do not do places them at risk of acquiring chronic diseases or experiencing serious injuries.

The behavioral components associated with the modern pattern of disease and injury create the potential for preventing most of these health problems by changing behavior. Comprehensive health promotion and education programs provide the foundation for modern disease prevention.

Ideally, the health promotion and education process begins early. Early education provides the opportunity to reach children and youth before they begin to adopt the behaviors associated with chronic disease, sexually transmitted disease, drug use, injury and mental illness. Through a systematic review of health promotion and disease prevention, educators can help children and youth enhance their health while helping them avoid illness and injury.

The *Health Facts* Series

Fitness: Health Facts is part of a series designed to provide clear, concise content and to be complementary to curricula published by ETR Associates and other health education curricula. Other volumes in this series that relate to the topic of fitness include *Nutrition and Body Image, Self-Esteem and Mental Health, Disease* and *Injury Prevention.*

Classroom teachers, counselors, school nurses and others are often called upon to become instant health educators. They may be asked to answer questions, present information and lead discussions on health topics in which they feel unprepared.

The *Health Facts* series is designed to be a handy reference for individuals who would like additional background information on particular health topics. The emphasis is on topics and examples that are relevant to youth of middle and high school age. References and resource listings direct the reader to additional relevant information. All of the volumes in this series offer a user-friendly format that is easy to read and factual.

The volumes discuss health and disease in straightforward language. Educators may want to review each volume for its appropriateness for their school and community before assigning the books for student use.

This book and the rest of the series can serve as useful additions to classroom, school or library collections. Health care professionals may choose individual volumes or the entire series as a convenient reference for patient education programs or as reading material in office waiting rooms. Individuals may find the series useful as a home reference as well.

Why Be Physically Fit?

Myth: With exercise, if there's no pain, there's no gain.

Fact: New research shows that it is not necessary to suffer in order to be healthy. Significant health benefits can be gained from moderate exercise each day. In fact, pain during exercise may be a sign of problems that shouldn't be overlooked.

Physical fitness is essential to good health. Fitness is a combination of qualities that enable an individual to meet the physical demands of daily life and still have energy left for other activities.

Health-related physical fitness is characterized by the ability to perform daily activities with vigor and the demonstration of traits that are linked to low risk of diseases such as heart disease. Becoming physically fit requires some type of regular physical activity, along with other healthful habits such as a healthy diet.

Age, heredity and behavior all influence the level of a person's fitness. Age and heredity are beyond individual control, and people vary in their capacity for physical fitness. However, all people can improve their level of fitness by the choices they make every day. Fitness continually changes in response to health behaviors such as physical activity and diet.

Benefits of Being Physically Fit

There is broad agreement that being physically fit makes a person feel good. Physically fit individuals can tolerate stress better and maintain longer periods of mental alertness. Getting regular exercise that improves fitness also helps a person stay healthy.

One major benefit of exercise is that people who increase their physical activity are more likely to adopt other lifestyle habits that further lower their risks of both cancer and cardiovascular disease. People who exercise are also likely to eat less, to cope more effectively with stress and even to quit an established smoking habit. These changes can create a synergistic effect, in which the benefits build upon one another to improve health and further lower the risks of disease.

In short, the benefits of being physically fit are many. Physical fitness can result in the following advantages:

- longer lifespan
- physiological improvements
- psychological and psychosocial benefits

Benefits to Life Expectancy

Recent research shows that people who are physically fit are less likely to die early than those who lead a sedentary life. A study of more than thirteen thousand men and women found a strong and consistent inverse relationship between physical fitness and death rates. That is, the more physically fit a person was, the less likely he or she was to die of any cause. The more sedentary a person was, the more likely she or he was to die of all causes.

A very important finding was that the levels of fitness that were found to be protective were moderate levels that are attainable by most adults. The lower death rates in the more fit individuals were mostly due to lower risks of cancer and cardiovascular disease. The study found that if all the unfit persons became fit, the death rates could be expected to drop by 9% for men and by more than 15% for women.

Life Expectancy and Exercise...Food for Thought

A question to ponder: Person A leads an active lifestyle from the age of about twenty years on, while Person B does not. Assuming their lifestyles are identical in all other ways, will Person A outlive Person B, and if so, by how much?

a. Person A will not necessarily outlive Person B.
b. Person A will outlive Person B by about two years.
c. Person A will outlive Person B by about four years.
d. Person A will outlive Person B by about eight years.
e. Person A will outlive Person B by about eleven years.

The answer is "b"—an active person will outlive an inactive person by an average of about two years.

In response to the study in the *New England Journal of Medicine* that reported this information, a cardiologist sent in his own calculations. He had calculated that depending on exercise intensity, the amount of time it would take to do the amount of exercise needed to extend life by two years would come to...two years! "Thus, the bad news is that although you may live an extra two years, those two years will be spent jogging," he wrote.

Clearly, if the two years are spent doing activities that are pleasurable or purposeful (and for some jogging may fit into this category), then it would be a worthwhile trade-off.

Adapted from B. Stamford and P. Shimer. 1990. *Fitness without exercise.* New York: Warner Books.

Physiological Benefits

Exercise strengthens muscle and bone. It works the circulatory and respiratory systems, so they deliver needed amounts of food and oxygen to the cells with less effort. Exercise also helps to develop coordination, balance and reaction time, which help people conduct everyday activities.

Physiological benefits gained through exercise include the following:

- stronger heart
- lower blood pressure
- increased metabolism
- longevity and positive changes in the aging process
- oxygen delivery
- healthier immune system

■ **Stronger heart:** With regular exercise, the heart can pump much more blood each minute than the heart of an inactive person. Its action becomes more mechanically efficient. More oxygen can be transported to the muscles, and the muscles can perform efficiently for a longer period of time.

In a person who is physically fit, the resting pulse becomes slower. After exercising or experiencing emotional stress, the increases in pulse rate are less than they were before physical conditioning. This pulse-lowering effect may offer some protection against heart attacks, which often are precipitated by a rapid pulse rate. Most experts believe sudden heart attack death is due to a rapid and ineffective heart action.

Some of the cardiovascular protection from exercise may come from beneficial changes in fats, or *lipids,* in the blood. These changes include decreases in *low-density* and *very low-density lipoproteins,* the cholesterol in the blood that produces *atherosclerosis,* or hardening of the arteries. Regular exercise also causes increases in the *high-density lipoproteins,* the cholesterol in the blood that is associated with lowered cardiovascular death rates.

- **Lower blood pressure:** The blood pressure of people who exercise regularly is about 35% lower than the blood pressure of people who are inactive. Together with other behavioral changes such as salt restriction, weight reduction and stress control, exercise is used as treatment for high blood pressure.

- **Increased metabolism:** Metabolism is the process by which the body uses food to release energy and uses the energy to build and repair body tissues. The more a person exercises, the more calories are burned. Regular vigorous exercise also seems to curb the appetite. It can prevent the development of diabetes or lessen its severity.

- **Longevity and positive changes in the aging process:** These are additional benefits of regular exercise. With age, muscle mass tends to decrease and the percentage of body fat increases. Often bones lose calcium and become brittle. Muscle strength declines, and blood pressure can increase. The amount of blood that the heart can pump gets smaller. The chest wall becomes stiffer, breathing capacity decreases, and oxygen delivery decreases as a result.

  Regular exercise can reverse many of these changes. Heart and lung capacities can increase, and blood pressure can become lower. With increased fitness, muscle strength increases and body fat decreases. Reaction time can also improve and reflexes become faster. Improvements in bone strength can help protect against *osteoporosis,* a disease that results in loss of bone density and poor bone strength.

- **Oxygen delivery:** Use of oxygen in the body improves through exercise. These changes improve the ability of the muscles to generate energy.

- **Healthier immune system:** Some research suggests that the extra *endorphins* (chemicals that act as natural painkillers in the body) produced by the brain during vigorous exercise can increase immune system activity. With exercise, body temperature rises. Elevated body temperature has been linked to improvements in immune activity.

Psychological and Psychosocial Benefits

There seems to be a strong association between fitness and psychological well-being. Exercise is a good way to release tension. Studies indicate that people who exercise regularly are less tired, more relaxed, more productive at work, more satisfied with their appearance and more self-confident.

Some key psychological and psychosocial benefits of regular exercise include:

- stress reduction
- higher self-esteem
- reduction in or prevention of depression
- social benefits

- **Stress reduction:** Vigorous exercise is an important tool in managing stress. Stress can appear as tension, anxiety or a pounding heart. Other signs of stress include difficulty falling asleep, compulsive eating and perspiring heavily.

  Reasons exercise is effective in managing stress include:
  - It temporarily removes a person from the stressors of daily life.
  - It improves an individual's mood. Exercise produces relaxation and feelings of confidence in one's abilities.
  - Exercising provides an opportunity to think out problems and work out feelings.

  However, when exercise becomes an obsession, it can actually result in increased stress levels. In extreme cases, anticipation of excessively strenuous exercise routines can raise stress levels and have negative effects on health.

- **Higher self-esteem:** Self-esteem can be enhanced by mastering exercise goals that earlier seemed impossible to meet. Improvements in coordination, muscle tone, posture and complexion help people feel good about themselves.

- **Reduction in or prevention of depression:** Depression often is associated with a lack of physical and mental activity. Exercise has been found to be a useful way to counter mild depression. Endorphins are produced in greater quantity during exercise, and this increased production may cause improvements in mood, appetite and even memory.

- **Social benefits:** Activities can be solitary or social. When activities are done with family or friends, bonds can be strengthened and companionship enjoyed.

Some Ways to Get a Workout— And Improve Relationships at Home

Some ways people miss out on burning calories around the house:

- Neglecting to help bring groceries in from the car. Depending on the size of the purchase and carrying distance, about fifteen to thirty calories are involved. This is enough for a weight gain of about a pound if avoided three times a week for a year.
- Failing to help with kitchen cleanup. In fifteen minutes of cleaning up, about forty calories are spent. If avoided once each day, this could cost about four pounds a year.
- Shouting from a sitting position rather than getting up and going to find the person. As many as three calories are retained that could be burned each time this occurs—enough for a weight gain of more than a pound of fat if done five times a day for a year.

Source: B. Stamford and P. Shimer. 1990. *Fitness without exercise.* New York: Warner Books.

The Fitness Crisis

Despite the recognized value of physical activity, exercise levels of Americans have not significantly improved. It is estimated that more than a quarter of a million deaths each year in the United States are due to lack of regular physical activity—a "sedentary" lifestyle. This lack of exercise contributes to high cholesterol levels and high blood pressure, among other health problems. In 1986, it was found that less than 10% of the U.S. adult population actually exercised at the recommended levels. In fact, fully 24% of adults were completely sedentary.

Fewer than half of American children get enough exercise for minimal levels of fitness. Forty percent of children between the ages of five and eight show at least one major risk factor for heart disease, such as elevated serum cholesterol, high blood pressure or obesity. Not only are schools not providing the needed programs, but students do not have the role models they need for fitness at home.

Among ethnic minority populations, older persons and those with lower incomes or levels of education, the picture is even bleaker. Participation in regular physical activity remains low. In fact, socioeconomic class is consistently the strongest predictor of exercise; blue-collar working men are among the least likely to engage in regular exercise programs. While 37% of professionals state that they exercise regularly, only 8% of unskilled working persons say that they do so.

Some blue-collar jobs provide more physical activity opportunities on the job site than other types of jobs. But research shows that despite this fact, blue-collar workers suffer more from heart attacks, strokes and high blood pressure than more sedentary white-collar workers. Health habits away from the job appear to be part of the reason.

For many Americans, dependence upon technology is one enticement to inactivity. For example, people who live in suburbs or similar types of communities often spend much of their time driving. Increased use of computers at businesses and at home can tend to produce a sedentary lifestyle unless a conscious effort is made to get exercise.

But the biggest influence on fitness and recreation patterns has been television. American children of school age watch an average of 24 hours of television each week, and adults watch even more. This sedentary type of recreation often takes the place of physical activity. For many, watching television is also a stimulus for eating unhealthy foods in a habitual way.

A New Approach to Fitness

Some researchers have proposed that the "failure" of the fitness movement in terms of public health is partly due to an overemphasis on high-intensity exercise. In the past, it was thought that for physical fitness to have a positive effect on health, people needed to perform "vigorous" physical activity (such as jogging) for periods of twenty minutes or longer three to five times a week. This was the "no pain, no gain" approach.

Research on exercise habits shows that most people who begin a three-workout-a-week exercise program don't stick to it for more than a few months. For many, the time required for such a workout is impractical and can't be sustained. It may be perceived as an unaffordable luxury. And sitting on a stationary bicycle or at a rowing machine may seem more like a punishment than a health effort.

Now, health experts say that it is not necessary to suffer in order to be healthy. Several studies have shown that many health benefits can be gained from moderate exercise, which includes many types of activity in a person's daily life—from housework to gardening. A little physical activity can reduce the risk of disease as much as quitting smoking can.

According to the U.S. Centers for Disease Control and Prevention (CDC) and the American College of Sports Medicine, accumulating thirty minutes or more of moderate physical activity over the course of most days of the week is an effective way to improve health. Since the time doesn't have to be spent all at once to be beneficial, it is possible to do activities that take only a few minutes, as long as there are enough of them over the course of the day to add up. Activities such as walking up stairs, gardening, raking leaves, doing laundry or walking can be "counted," along with planned exercise or recreation such as swimming or cycling.

The Pleasure Principle

Researchers now believe that it is better to manage one's health with less effort and more fun—and that by doing so, health will be enriched and not just maintained. They point out that through evolution, health-promoting acts are biologically connected with positive feelings or pleasure. Vitality and good health seem to come not only from good health habits, but also from a positive state of mind. This state of mind has been called the "pursuit of healthy pleasures."

These researchers emphasize the need to restore "sensibility" to the pursuit of health. They note that worrying too much about anything—calories and cholesterol included—is not good for health, and that living optimistically, with pleasure and zest, is good for health. This is not to say that calories and cholesterol are not important, but rather that obsessing over them may not be the best approach. They should be kept in perspective.

Moderate Activity as a Way to Fitness

"No pain, no gain" is an outdated concept. To be healthy, exercise doesn't require burdensome regimes. Every bit of activity counts toward achieving better health. While contemporary life in the United States has become too sedentary, the fitness formulas of the 1970s and 1980s were an overreaction. It actually takes very little physical activity to achieve many health benefits.

In a well-known study of nearly seventeen thousand Harvard graduates, health benefits began for those who burned up as few as five hundred calories a week. That could be achieved by a 15-minute walk each day, two hours of bowling or even a one-hour squash game each week. Even with such a modest level of activity, death rates declined by 20%.

While modest health benefits can come from five hundred calories a week of physical activity, this level is not enough to help avoid heart attack. According to a study from Stanford University, a minimum of 1,050 calories per week of physical activity is needed to decrease heart disease risk. Additional research shows that for cardiovascular health, the preferred range is from the minimum of 1,050 calories to an optimum of 2,000 calories per week.

Evidence from many more studies shows that people who are physically inactive have about twice the rate of heart disease and heart attacks as more active people. Complete physical inactivity is about as risky as cigarette smoking, high blood pressure and high cholesterol.

Another reason to emphasize more moderate exercise is that strenuous exercise can cause injuries. Each year, 20% of all joggers who run ten miles a week are injured severely enough to have to cut back on their exercise. For those who run thirty miles, the injury rate rises to 40%. As one analysis concluded, "The tortoise who keeps a steady pace is more likely to pass the running rabbits nursing their injured feet, knees, and backs on the side of the road" (Ornstein and Sobel, 1989).

Very high levels of exercise can also be harmful to women's reproductive systems. Some women may not ovulate, or they may miss menstrual periods. Hormone levels can drop, which may increase the risk of osteoporosis.

Fitness and Weight Control

According to laws of biochemistry and physics, calories burned by doing heavy activity count no more than those burned by doing light activity. Light activity may even be better for weight loss if it is engaged in more frequently—and especially after eating.

In addition, when fat is burned as fuel, it comes from storage areas all over the body, no matter which muscles are active. The way to trim specific areas of the body is to trim down all over, which can be done without doing monotonous and time-consuming exercises.

Condensing all of one's daily physical activity into one intense workout is less effective for weight control than seizing all opportunities during the day for activity, no matter how small. Some examples include taking "mini-walks"—such as taking trips up or down stairs, down the hall or down the block—walking the dog, washing the car, going shopping, mowing the lawn, stacking firewood or unloading groceries from the car.

Timing of Exercise

A physiological phenomenon called the *thermic effect of food* is also relevant to weight control. After a meal, the body's metabolic rate goes up by about 10% as a result of the processes it requires to get the meal digested. This 10% can be almost doubled if light physical activity is undertaken while the digestive processes are still going on.

When this happens, food "burns hotter," in a sense, with fewer calories made available for fat storage as a result. This phenomenon suggests that it may be advantageous to undertake light activity such as walking or doing yardwork within about half an hour of eating moderately.

Exercise shortly before eating can accomplish the same effect. A greater "caloric burn" from a meal is created when exercise precedes eating.

Dietary Changes

Today the average American weighs about 10% more than in 1910. Yet, the average American doesn't consume more calories than in 1910. So what accounts for the difference?

Reduced physical activity is only part of the problem. Although Americans now are more sedentary, significant dietary changes over the past eighty years have had a major influence, as well. These changes include:

- Intake of dietary fat has risen by about 15%.
- Intake of refined sugar has increased by about 20%.
- Instead of eating small, evenly spaced meals throughout the day, Americans tend to eat larger, more-infrequent meals each day.

Some recent research indicates that calories from fat are much more likely to convert to body fat than calories from carbohydrates or protein. In other words, most body fat starts as dietary fat.

Eating smaller and more-frequent meals has been found to help with weight control. Large meals call up large amounts of insulin, which encourages calories to be stored as fat rather than burned. Also, large meals tend to make people feel drowsy and less inclined to do anything physical. For these reasons, skipping meals during the day and sitting down to a large evening meal will actually thwart weight loss efforts.

Another problem is that many Americans eat for reasons other than hunger. External cues may have confused the natural ability to regulate food intake. For example, infants eat in response to body hunger cues and stop eating in response to feelings of *satiety* (a feeling of fullness and satisfaction). But later on, external cues such as watching television or internal cues other than hunger (such as stress or unmet emotional needs) may trigger a desire to eat. A combination of these conditions is conducive to weight gain that cannot be managed by increases in activity alone.

Thus, fitness requires not only regular physical activity, but also a healthy diet. According to some experts, dietary fat is the real culprit in most weight problems and cardiovascular problems in the United States. They advocate "lipo-fitness," not just aerobic fitness, as an effective way to improve overall health.

Currently, the average American gets 40% of dietary calories from fat. A diet that yields only 20% of calories from fat can result in body fat loss without any cutback on total calories. This effect occurs because instead of getting the calories from fat, the calories are obtained from foods that are not only highly nutritious but also raise the body's metabolic rate. Such foods include lowfat protein sources and, to some extent, complex carbohydrates. This effect can be further boosted with moderate exercise around the time of eating.

Current government guidelines recommend a reduction in calories from fat from 40% to 30% and an increase in complex carbohydrates from about 20% of calories to about 50% of calories. These are only guidelines—a goal to aim for. But any steps toward reducing the proportion of fat in the diet, along with increasing the complex carbohydrates, would be an improvement that could show some tangible results.

The best approach to weight control couples increased physical activity with dietary changes. Making moderate improvements in both areas can enhance fitness and health.

1-Minute Facts

- Physical fitness is a combination of qualities that enable an individual to meet the physical demands of daily life and still have energy left for other interests.

- People can improve their level of fitness by the choices they make every day.

- Several studies have indicated that moderate exercise, attained from many types of activity in daily life, can offer many health benefits.

- One major benefit of exercise is that people who increase their physical activity are more likely to adopt other lifestyle habits that further lower their risk of disease.

- The benefits of physical fitness include longer lifespan, physiological improvements and psychological and psychosocial benefits.

- Exercise benefits the heart, blood pressure, metabolism, longevity and aging processes, oxygen delivery and use, and the immune system.

- Psychological and psychosocial benefits of regular exercise include stress reduction, enhanced self-esteem, less depression and social benefits.

- Fitness requires a healthy diet as well as regular physical activity.

- Dietary guidelines suggest reducing daily fat intake from 40% to 30% of calories.

THE ELEMENTS OF FITNESS

MYTH: If a person stops exercising regularly, his or her muscle turns to fat.

Fact: Muscle and fat are specialized tissues that perform separate functions and are not interchangeable. Exercise increases the size of muscles. Eating an excess amount of calories without enough exercising increases the size of fat cells.

Physical fitness is the ability of the heart, blood vessels, lungs and muscles to function at their best. A person who is physically fit can handle physical, intellectual, social and emotional challenges without undue fatigue. Exercise, rest, sleep and good nutrition are all required for fitness. Fitness has the following key components:

- cardiorespiratory endurance
- body composition
- flexibility
- muscular strength
- muscular endurance

Cardiorespiratory Endurance

Cardiorespiratory endurance, or *aerobic fitness*, is the foundation for whole-body fitness. It refers to the body's ability to take in and use oxygen so the muscles can function. The level of cardiorespiratory endurance depends on the ability of the heart muscle and lungs to supply oxygen to the cells in the body and the ability of the cells to use the oxygen efficiently and to eliminate carbon dioxide.

Most experts agree that cardiorespiratory endurance is the most important element of fitness. In studies designed to measure fitness and its relationship to health, cardiorespiratory endurance is usually what is measured.

Engaging in aerobic types of exercise on a regular basis is the best way to enhance cardiorespiratory endurance. Aerobic exercise requires the skeletal muscles, heart, vascular system and lungs to work hard for prolonged periods. In response, these muscles become stronger and able to work hard for progressively longer amounts of time. Aerobic exercise includes walking, swimming, running, cycling and cross-country skiing.

HISTORICAL NOTE: REGULAR EXERCISE

In the early 1960s, less than 5% of the adult population in the United States engaged in regular aerobic exercise. Despite all of the fitness promotion since that time, the 1990 Youth Risk Behavior survey conducted by the Centers for Disease Control and Prevention found that 50% of male and 75% of female high school students polled did not exercise on a regular basis (three or more times per week).

During intense aerobic exercise, the heart rate can rise as much as 400%, increasing the amount of blood pumped from five quarts a minute to as many as twenty quarts a minute. Regular aerobic exercise builds the heart's endurance by strengthening and thickening the walls of the pumping chamber, which increases the amount of blood pumped with each heartbeat.

Sometimes people undertake activities that require a level of intensity that outstrips the body's ability to transport oxygen efficiently to the muscles. When the oxygen demands of the muscles cannot be met, a situation called *oxygen debt* occurs. Activity that continues past the point when oxygen debt begins will require a type of energy production that does not depend on oxygen.

This oxygen-deprived form of energy production is called *anaerobic* (without oxygen) energy production. This type of energy is needed for many intense, short-duration activities, such as weight lifting or sprinting. These activities quickly cause muscle fatigue.

Activities that are usually considered aerobic, such as walking, cycling or jogging, can become anaerobic when they are either increased in intensity or continued for an extended period. Marathon runners, distance swimmers and cyclists have highly developed aerobic fitness; they take in, transport and use oxygen in a highly efficient manner. For this reason, they can continue their activity over a long period of time without becoming fatigued.

WHEN AEROBIC BECOMES ANAEROBIC

When exercise gets too intense, more energy is produced by using the stored glycogen in muscles. This is an anaerobic process, and lactic acid starts accumulating in the blood. Carbon dioxide is produced, and breathing becomes labored. Labored breathing and discomfort from the increased acidity are signs that the threshold from aerobic to anaerobic has been crossed.

Factors Affecting Aerobic Fitness

Currently, cardiovascular diseases (heart attack, stroke, atherosclerosis) are the leading cause of death for Americans. Research shows that improving aerobic capacity can help reduce the risk of developing these diseases. Aerobic fitness levels are also influenced by factors other than training. These factors include:

- heredity
- gender
- age
- body fat

■ **Heredity** plays a significant role in aerobic fitness potential. It is thought to be responsible for about 40% of aerobic fitness potential. Individuals inherit a number of characteristics that contribute to aerobic fitness, such as lung capacity, heart size, amount of red blood cells and hemoglobin, capillary supply, and types of muscle fibers.

■ **Gender** is related to aerobic fitness only after puberty. Women average about three-fourths of men's aerobic capacity. One reason may be that men tend to have more hemoglobin in their blood. Women also have more body fat—25% for college-age women compared with 12.5% for college-age men. Women also are generally smaller and have less muscle mass.

In the past, women did not compete in races longer than the half mile. However, today, among the top endurance athletes of the world, aerobic fitness and performance differences between women and men are diminishing.

- **Age:** Aerobic fitness usually increases through the late teens or early twenties, then slowly declines over time. Inactive people lose 8% to 10% per decade, while those who remain physically active can cut the decline in half. Despite the typical decline in aerobic fitness with age, improvements can be made at all ages.

- **Body fat** increases are thought to be responsible for about half of the decline in aerobic fitness that comes with age. Since aerobic fitness is measured by dividing oxygen consumption by body weight, the easiest way to improve is through weight loss. Thus, weight loss alone can improve aerobic fitness, without any exercise at all.

Body Composition

Body composition refers to the proportion of body fat to lean tissue. Body composition is usually expressed as the percentage of body weight that is fat. As a person becomes more physically fit, the percentage of fat tissue decreases and the percentage of lean tissue increases.

Lean tissue includes muscle, bone, cartilage, connective tissue, nerves, skin and internal organs. The amount of muscle and size of bones are the factors that most strongly influence the proportion of the body that is lean tissue.

The body needs a certain amount of fat to survive. Fat stores certain nutrients and converts them into energy, provides insulation for the body and protects internal organs. The body uses fat tissue every day.

But excess body fat can increase the risk of many diseases, including heart disease, diabetes and certain cancers. The location of fat on the body is also important. Fat around the abdomen (the "apple" shape) represents more of a health risk than fat that accumulates elsewhere, such as on the hips and buttocks (the "pear" shape).

The number of fat cells a person has is determined at a very young age. While fat cells can become smaller, they cannot be lost. Females have more stored fat in their bodies than males.

Although too much body fat may be a health concern, cultural beliefs about "ideal" body composition can complicate the issue. In American society, the ideal body type promoted by the mass media depicts unrealistically low body-fat levels. In reality, ideal body composition differs substantially from person to person and may have a strong genetic base. Promoting one ideal image ignores the basic facts that human beings have a variety of sizes and shapes and that this diversity is positive.

Body composition, size of bones and muscle structure are influenced by heredity as well as by diet and fitness. Generally, people inherit a tendency toward one of three body types: a type that is tall and thin *(ectomorph)*, a type that is muscular and of average height *(mesomorph)*, and a type that is short and rounded *(endomorph)*.

Flexibility

Flexibility is the ability of joints to move through a full range of possible motion. Movement at the joints allows people to bend, touch their toes or rotate their bodies. When a person is flexible, the body does not get stiff easily. Flexibility makes it less likely that muscles will become injured or that lower back pain will develop.

Flexibility depends on the elasticity of the muscles and connective tissues (tendons and ligaments) and the condition of the joints. If flexibility is maintained, the body can move and bend instead of becoming injured in response to movements.

The range of motion increases when joints and muscles are warmed up. Stretching exercises are most successful after some warm-up but before vigorous exercise begins. Stretching during a cool-down period after exercise can help reduce muscle soreness. Flexibility exercises are important when training for strength or endurance because they help maintain the range of motion. Even after years of participating in an activity, muscles can become tight and sore. Daily stretching can help make an activity more enjoyable.

Flexibility is influenced by gender, with females being more flexible than males. Age, posture and amount of fat and muscle also play a part. Generally, people become more flexible until adolescence, when levels of flexibility start to decline.

People who are inactive are less flexible than those who enjoy a variety of activities requiring movement. Active people stretch their muscles more than inactive people do. When most of the day is spent sitting, muscles connected to the knee, hip and elbow joints start to shorten. Muscles must be stretched in order to remain flexible. Ballet and gymnastics are examples of activities that require great flexibility.

Muscular Strength

Muscular strength is the ability of the muscles to work. It is the amount of force they can exert when they contract. Muscle strength is needed for all movement, which is created by the contraction of specific muscle groups.

Strong muscles enable the body to move more efficiently and do more work. They also help support and protect other body structures, such as joints and internal organs. Through exercise, systematically requiring muscles to do more and more work, muscle strength can be increased.

Factors Influencing Strength

Muscular strength varies according to gender and the types of muscle fiber a person has.

- **Gender:** Until age 12 to 14, boys and girls have approximately equal muscular strength. After this point, on the average, males have greater muscular strength. One reason for the difference may be the increase in the male sex hormone *testosterone* at puberty. The average male has ten times the testosterone of an average female, and testosterone is an *anabolic* (growth-inducing) steroid that helps muscles enlarge. Muscle size is associated with strength. However, it could also be that having more of this hormone makes a person more aggressive and willing to train harder.

  Body fat may also contribute to the differences. Young women have twice the percentage of body fat of young men. When strength is measured per unit of lean body weight (body weight minus fat weight), the differences start to diminish. In fact, women tend to have slightly stronger legs, but weaker arms. As more women engage in occupations requiring upper body strength, such as police work, firefighting or construction, as well as sports, women's average arm strength may approach that of men.

- **Types of muscle fiber:** There are two types of muscle fiber—slow twitch and fast twitch. Fast twitch fibers are larger and have more potential for the development of tension. People with more of these types of fibers have greater potential for the development of muscular strength. The type of muscle fiber a person has is partly due to heredity.

Muscular Endurance

Muscular endurance is the ability of the muscle to sustain an activity or continue to perform work. It is the ability to persist, to have stamina. Like muscular strength, endurance is necessary for everyday tasks, such as mowing the lawn or playing basketball. Endurance is often the key to success in a sport, since repetition leads to skill, and repetition requires endurance.

Training increases the number of capillaries in the muscles, so that the muscles can receive more blood during exercise. The activity of enzymes, certain chemicals in the muscles, also increases with exercise. Enzymes allow muscles to extract and use oxygen more efficiently, thus improving muscular endurance.

The Importance of Diet

A person's diet can directly influence muscle endurance. Research has shown that the best endurance comes from a high carbohydrate diet. A high carbohydrate diet is good for endurance as well as for general fitness and health. The diet recommended by exercise physiologists, who study the effects of exercise on the body and the relationship of activity and fitness to health, includes:

- 25% of calories from fat
- 15% of calories from protein
- 60% of calories from complex carbohydrates

Complex carbohydrates are an excellent source of energy and include other nutrients and fiber. Some examples of complex carbohydrates are corn, rice, beans, potatoes and whole grain products (cereals, breads and pasta).

Historical Note: Taking Fitness Seriously

The physiology of fitness began to receive serious scientific attention in the 1950s. Studies of British bus drivers and civil servants showed a link between regular exercise and a lower risk of heart disease.

Before that time, fitness was of interest mainly for military preparedness. During the two world wars and the Korean War, U.S. military leaders became concerned about the fitness levels of draftees. They called for greater attention to fitness in the schools.

Today, fitness is valued for its relationship to health as well as for its contributions to performance in work and sport.

1-Minute Facts

- The key components of fitness are cardiorespiratory endurance, or aerobic fitness, body composition, flexibility, muscular strength and muscular endurance.
- Cardiorespiratory endurance is the body's ability to take in and use oxygen so that the muscles can function.
- Body composition refers to the proportion of body fat to lean tissue.
- Flexibility is the ability of joints to move through a full range of possible motion.
- Muscular strength is the ability of the muscles to work.
- Muscular endurance is the ability of the muscle to sustain an activity or continue to perform work.

Assessing Fitness Levels

Myth: The only purpose of a diet is to lose weight.

Fact: Diet is the kind and amount of food regularly consumed. Special diets may be used to lose, gain or maintain weight; reduce health risks; or cure or alleviate illness.

Increasing evidence that a high level of fitness isn't necessary to achieve the health benefits of exercise has led the U.S. Department of Health and Human Service to change its objectives for the nation for the year 2000. The new objectives emphasize reducing inactivity and increasing light to moderate activity. The previous set of objectives, published for the year 1990, emphasized more intense activity and fitness.

In evaluating an individual's level of fitness, a few considerations should be kept in mind. First, the way that fitness is measured will depend on the purpose of the measurement. If the aim is to assess whether there is enough daily activity to lower health risks, including risk of heart disease, then assessing all types of daily activity—the overall pattern—is the best approach. If the aim is to achieve aerobic fitness or to enhance muscular strength, then specific tests can be used to assess fitness in these areas.

However, since the capacity for fitness is influenced by genetic makeup, individual fitness should be evaluated on individual capacity, not by comparison with others. In other words, progress toward fitness should involve competition with oneself, not others.

Similarly, it must be recognized that there is a range of body types and sizes, which cannot always be changed through behavior. Understanding individual fitness levels involves an awareness of individual capacity for fitness and an acceptance of differences in body type that may or may not be amenable to change.

Weight Control and Body Image

Americans usually think that being healthy means being thin. But the truth is that people who are of average weight or slightly overweight are actually the healthiest. People who are either very lean or very obese face the greatest health risks.

When Is Fat Unhealthy?

People who have diabetes, high blood pressure, high cholesterol, heart disease or back pain may need to be concerned about weight control. People who are 40% above their desirable weight, according to actuarial tables, may find that weight reduction has health benefits. Someone who tends to "yo-yo," losing weight and then gaining it back (or gaining back even more), may derive more health benefits by maintaining a stable weight. While diet is crucial to health, "dieting" is not a healthy way to eat.

Where the fat is carried on the body may also affect health risks. Fat around the middle of the body is linked with diabetes and heart disease. Fat carried in the hips and thighs appears to be less hazardous to health. From a health perspective, it is fortunate that fat around the waistline seems to be easier to shed.

It has been shown that small changes in people who are significantly overweight (at least 60% above ideal weight) can produce fairly large improvements to health. For example, one study showed that after losing only 10% of their weight, 40% of those with high blood pressure could discontinue their medications and one-third of those with adult-onset diabetes could be weaned off their insulin.

Cultural Meanings of Fat

In truth, except for the really obese, Americans' fear of fat is related more to appearance than to health. In assessing fitness, the cultural ideal of thinness should be separated from the reality of a "healthy weight." Some researchers point out that getting fatter signifies getting (and looking) older, since it is common to gain weight with age.

In fact, in some parts of the world, being fat is considered a sign of wealth and prestige. While young people may be slim and athletic, adults are expected to be heavy as a sign of their maturity and status in the community. In the more youth-oriented American society, people often want to lose weight for cosmetic rather than health reasons.

Fitness and Body Image

The mental image people have of their bodies is called *body image*. The choice to improve or maintain fitness is influenced by body image. While many people have features that they believe need improvement or that they dislike, only some of these features can be changed through personal behavior.

Basically, people have two choices regarding the physical features they don't like (such as height) that cannot be changed:

- They can refuse to accept the body as it is and continue to feel bad about it.
- They can change the way they think and feel about those features.

Many physical characteristics are amenable to change, although the amount of change possible may depend on other factors such as heredity. To improve these characteristics, such as muscular strength, specific assessment tests and workout plans can be undertaken.

Exploring Body Image Issues

Below are some questions to ponder about body image. There are no right or wrong answers, but exploring your responses to them can lead to personal resolutions for change and self-improvement.

- Am I dissatisfied with my body size and shape?
- Do I talk about my unhappiness with my body?
- Am I always on a diet or going on a diet?
- Do I express guilt when I eat certain foods, or do I refuse to eat certain foods while commenting that I am dieting to lose weight?
- Do I make negative comments about other people's sizes and shapes? Do I feel superior to them because I think my body is better than theirs?
- Am I prejudiced against people who are overweight? Do I avoid making friends with overweight people? Am I embarrassed to be seen in public with overweight people?

Source: J. Ikeda and P. Naworski. 1992. *Am I Fat? Helping Young Children Accept Differences in Body Size.* Santa Cruz, CA: ETR Associates.

Assessing Overall Activity Level

In assessing fitness, a first step is to evaluate daily activity levels. However, the specifics of each assessment will vary depending on age and gender. Basic activity "tests" have been devised by a number of experts. Completing a general fitness inventory can indicate whether people are more fit than they may think. A high activity score suggests that additional workouts are not needed for health. Lower scores indicate that more activity is desirable for long-term health benefits.

The following test helps evaluate activity levels for youth ages 12 to 18. It can be used as a guide in setting activity goals.

Fitness Choice Inventory for Youth

Directions: Answer *yes* or *no* to the following questions. Give yourself the number of points indicated for each *yes* answer. Then add your points to determine your level of physical activity.

1. I usually walk at least 1 mile a day. (1 point) _____
2. I take the stairs instead of elevators or escalators. (1 point) _____
3. My daily routine involves:
   a. sitting at school or watching TV at home (0 points) _____
   b. some physical activity during or after school (4 points) _____
   c. several hours of heavy sports or work activity (8 points) _____
4. I ride my bike or walk instead of riding in a car. (1 point) _____
5. I do yard work or housework several hours each week. (2 points) _____
6. I dance at least once a week. (2 points) _____
7. I exercise when I'm feeling stressed. (2 points) _____
8. I do stretching exercises several times each week. (3 points) _____

9. Two or more times a week, I perform sit-ups, pull-ups or other exercises for at least ten minutes per session. (3 points) ____
10. I lift weights or use exercise equipment:
    a. about once a week (2 points) ____
    b. about twice a week (4 points) ____
    c. three times a week (7 points) ____
11. I engage in a vigorous fitness activity like jogging, aerobic dance or basketball (at least twenty continuous minutes per session):
    a. about once a week (3 points) ____
    b. about twice a week (5 points) ____
    c. at least three times per week (9 points) ____

Total points ____

Scoring:

0 to 7 points—Inactive. Becoming more active will help reduce your risk of health problems.

8 to 14 points—Moderately active. This amount of activity will help maintain or improve your present level of fitness.

15 to 25 points—Active. This amount of activity will maintain a good level of fitness.

26 points or more—Very active. This amount of activity will maintain a high level of fitness.

Adapted with permission from B. Hubbard. 1991. *Entering Adulthood: Moving into Fitness.* Santa Cruz, CA: ETR Associates.

Assessing Cardiorespiratory Endurance

Cardiorespiratory endurance—the capacity to take in, transport and use oxygen—is also called *aerobic fitness*. It can be measured in several ways. Some of the measurements are highly technical and require a laboratory or medical setting. Others can be done more simply with a minimum of equipment or technical know-how.

Technically, a laboratory test called the maximal oxygen consumption, or VO_2 max, has been considered the best way to measure cardiorespiratory endurance. A health risk assessment is usually completed first to ensure that taking the test will not be harmful to the person's health. The test involves using an electrocardiogram to measure heart rate and a special device to analyze metabolism while a person walks or runs on a treadmill.

During each minute the person is on the treadmill, the amount of oxygen consumed is computed as the test proceeds from low to high levels of aerobic effort. Scoring is reported as the amount of oxygen consumed per body weight. Because this type of test is expensive, time consuming and not readily available to most individuals, exercise physiologists recommend using less complicated methods of estimating aerobic fitness.

An Aerobic Fitness Test

Tests evaluating the ability to run are considered excellent indicators of aerobic fitness. They are considered to be the most suitable tests for active individuals, and they lend themselves well to group testing situations. The length of the run varies in different tests, but studies show that running tests lasting 12 minutes or more are best for assessing aerobic fitness. These are the tests most commonly used to assess cardiorespiratory endurance in children and youth.

Other types of tests, such as a step test, can also be used to measure aerobic capacity. The step test involves stepping on and off a step of a certain height for a measured amount of time. Fitness is assessed by determining the pulse rate after the stepping is completed.

ONE-MILE WALK/RUN TEST

A one-mile walk/run provides a simple field test of aerobic fitness. Participants should warm-up before the run, then rest. The run should be over a level measured course. Participants should be encouraged to maintain a constant pace, walking only if necessary. After running, cool-down activities such as walking and stretching should be done.

Runners should be timed. The following table shows average times for youth based on age and gender.

Age	Female	Male
12	11:00 min.	9:00 min.
13	10:30 min.	8:00 min.
14	10:30 min.	7:45 min.
15	10:30 min.	7:30 min.
16	10:30 min.	7:30 min.
17	10:30 min.	7:30 min.
18	10:30 min.	7:30 min.

A time faster than the average indicates a higher level of fitness, while a slower time indicates the need to improve fitness. The score can be used to set personal fitness goals and document the effects of training.

Adapted with permission from B. Hubbard. 1991. *Entering Adulthood: Moving into Fitness.* Santa Cruz, CA: ETR Associates.

Determining Body Composition

The body is made up of both fat tissue and lean tissue. Lean tissue comprises muscle, bone, skin, organs, etc. Body composition measures the proportion of each type that a person has. Heredity influences body composition as well as bone size and muscle structure. The type and frequency of physical activity engaged in also influences body composition. With exercise, the ratio of fat tissue to lean tissue changes. The percentage of fat tissue decreases, and the percentage of lean tissue increases.

Several methods can be used to determine body composition. The methods of measurement vary in degree of precision and in their practicality for the average person. Two of the most commonly used methods are *hydrostatic weighing* and *skinfold measurements.*

- **Hydrostatic weighing** is considered the "standard" for accuracy. This technique involves weighing a person both underwater and out of the water. The higher the weight in the water, the lower the percentage of body fat, and vice versa. Bone and muscle are more dense than fat, and they weigh more, so leaner people tend to sink and fatter people tend to float.

  However, this method requires expensive equipment and trained technicians, making it impractical for most people. Studies have shown that underwater weighing is subject to errors with certain people, especially those who are younger or older and those at extremes of leanness and fatness. Age-related differences in body water and bone density can throw the method off.

- **Skinfold measurements** offer a more practical method of providing a relatively accurate picture of body composition. The skinfold measure of body fat is based on the relationship of fat under the skin, or *subcutaneous fat,* to total body fat. Because one third of the body's fat may be located just under the skin, some carefully selected skinfold measurements can provide a fairly precise estimate of body fat.

Skinfold Measurement

Equipment needed: Skinfold calipers. Calipers need not be expensive to get accurate results.

Preparation: Participants should wear shorts and a short-sleeved shirt for the assessment.

Skinfold locations: Measurements should be taken at the triceps, midway between the elbow and the shoulder on the back of the arm, and the calf, just above the largest part of the calf on the inside of the leg.

Procedure: The skinfold should be grasped between the thumb and the index finger, and the calipers applied about one-half inch below the fingers. The calipers go in about as deep as the fold is wide. The measurement should be taken, the skinfold released, and the measurement repeated three times. Record the middle (median) score for each skinfold site.

Scoring: Add the triceps and calf scores to determine the final skinfold score. An average score for females ages 12 to 18 is 16 to 36 mm; for males ages 12 to 18, an average score is 12 to 25 mm. A score higher than average indicates a higher percentage of body fat; a lower score indicates a lower percentage of body fat. The score can be used to set personal fitness goals and document the effects of training.

Adapted with permission from B. Hubbard. 1991. *Entering Adulthood: Moving into Fitness.* Santa Cruz, CA: ETR Associates.

There is no such thing as "ideal" body composition. In the United States, the ideal body type promoted in the mass media usually depicts unrealistically low body-fat levels, especially for women but also for men. In reality, there is a spectrum of normal or appropriate percentages of body fat. The "right" proportion depends on many factors unique to each individual.

The appropriate proportion of body fat—fashion aside—is one that is consistent with optimal health over the lifespan. For women, a healthy range is between 22% and 35% of total weight: for men, between 12% and 25%. In the absence of heart disease, hypertension or diabetes, there is little health difference between the extremes at either end of the scale for both men and women.

Assessing Flexibility

Flexibility is the range of motion that the limbs are capable of. Skin, connective tissue, conditions within joints and excessive body fat can all restrict the range of motion. The more flexible a person's limbs are, the lower the potential for injury.

Lack of flexibility is involved in the development of many acute and chronic injuries and low-back problems. Everyone can benefit from regular stretching exercises, especially as connective tissue becomes less elastic with age.

Flexibility is influenced by gender, age, genes and current level of physical fitness. Assessing flexibility can be done with a simple test of hamstring flexibility.

Sit-and-Reach Test for Hamstring Flexibility

Equipment needed: yardstick and tape.

Preparation: Participants should prepare for the test by performing slow, sustained stretches of the low back and posterior thighs. The yardstick should be taped to the floor.

Procedure: Participants should sit with legs straight and heels about five inches apart, with the yardstick between the legs and the heels even with the 15-inch mark on the yardstick. Shoes should not be worn. While in a sitting position, participants should slowly stretch forward as far as possible.

Scoring: The score is the number of inches reached. An average score for youth under age 18, both male and female, is 25 cm or 10 inches (i.e., reaching to the 25-inch mark on the yardstick). The ability to reach farther than average suggests greater flexibility; reaching less far suggests less flexibility. The score can be used to set personal fitness goals and document the effects of training.

Adapted with permission from B. Hubbard. 1991. *Entering Adulthood: Moving into Fitness.* Santa Cruz, CA: ETR Associates.

Assessing Muscular Strength and Endurance

Various muscular fitness tests can be used to determine muscular strength and endurance, depending on the purpose. Typical ways muscular fitness is tested are by doing sit-ups (curl-ups), which test abdominal and lower back strength, and pull-ups, which assess upper body strength.

Testing Muscular Strength and Endurance

Abdominal and Lower Back Strength—Sit-Ups

Equipment needed: Mat or other comfortable surface and a stop watch or watch with a sweep second hand.

Procedure: Participants should lie flat on their backs with knees bent, shoulders touching the floor and arms extended above the thighs or by their sides, palms down. Feet should be flat on the floor, about 12 inches from the buttocks. Participants curl up by lifting the head and shoulders off the floor, sliding hands forward above the thighs or above the floor. They then curl down and repeat. The test starts when the timer indicates that timing has begun. After sixty seconds, performance is ended with the command to stop. Participants may rest between sit-ups, but the objective is to complete as many sit-ups as possible in sixty seconds.

Scoring: The score is the number of sit-ups completed in one minute. The following chart indicates average scores for youth based on age and gender.

Age	Female	Male
12	33	38
13	33	40
14	35	40
15	35	42
16	35	44
17	35	44
18	35	44

Upper Body Strength—Pull-Ups

Equipment needed: A horizontal metal or wooden bar about one and a half inches in diameter, high enough overhead to allow the body to hang without touching the floor.

Procedure: Participants begin by hanging from the bar with arms fully extended. They should grip the bar with an overhand grip. From the hanging position, the body is raised until the chin is over the bar. Participants should perform as many pull-ups as they can. There is no time limit.

Scoring: The score is the number of pull-ups performed. The following chart indicates average scores for youth based on age and gender.

Age	Female	Male
12	1	2
13	1	3
14	1	4
15	1	5
16	1	5
17	1	5
18	1	5

Scores higher than average indicate a greater level of fitness; lower scores indicate the need to improve fitness. The scores can be used to set personal fitness goals and document the effects of training.

Adapted with permission from B. Hubbard. 1991. *Entering Adulthood: Moving into Fitness.* Santa Cruz, CA: ETR Associates.

1-Minute Facts

- The new objectives for the nation for the year 2000 emphasize reducing inactivity and increasing light to moderate activity.

- Individual fitness should be evaluated on individual capacity, not by comparison with others.

- Specific assessment tests and exercise plans can improve fitness.

- Completing a general fitness inventory can help people assess their fitness.

- A running test can be used to measure aerobic fitness.

- Hydrostatic weighing and skinfold measurements are two of the methods most commonly used to determine body composition.

- Lack of flexibility is involved in the development of many acute and chronic injuries and low-back problems.

- Sit-ups and pull-ups can be used to assess muscular strength and endurance.

IMPROVING PHYSICAL FITNESS

MYTH: The main reason to exercise is to lose weight.

Fact: Exercise has long-term effects on a person's overall health, including blood pressure, metabolism, longevity, the immune system and stress levels. Benefits from physical fitness are physiological, psychological and social.

To improve overall fitness, health experts recommend accumulating thirty minutes or more of moderate-intensity physical activity during most days of the week. This recommendation is endorsed by the President's Council on Physical Fitness and the American Council of Sports Medicine.

This recommendation is based on the fact that it takes relatively little change in activity level to make a difference in long-term health. The important thing is to find ways to incorporate more activity into the day and to do so on a regular basis.

A more rigorous exercise program may also have benefits, but it may not be needed to improve health. An earlier recommendation was to get at least twenty minutes of continuous aerobic activity three to five days a week. While some Americans are able to adhere to such a schedule, many are not. Fortunately, moderate increases in daily activity level can improve health.

Not only does moderate exercise yield health benefits, it can also be a source of pleasure and provide a mental "time out." One key to being able to sustain a level of activity is to choose activities that are enjoyable or productive. Another strategy that works is to look for opportunities to include more physical activity in everyday tasks, such as taking the stairs instead of the elevator or parking at the far end of the parking lot and walking the extra distance.

Increasing Activity Level

People always expend energy, even when they are asleep, and expending energy means burning calories. A 150-pound person who is just sitting quietly uses about 75 calories each hour. This energy is needed by the heart and respiratory muscles for normal cellular metabolism and for maintaining body temperature. This use of calories while resting is called *basal metabolic rate.*

With movement, energy needs greatly increase. For example, a person who requires only a calorie a minute while resting can use more than twenty calories a minute during vigorous exercise. Walking expends about five calories a minute, jogging can burn ten or more, and running can require more than fifteen.

The calories burned during an activity will depend on body weight and intensity of effort. In general, a person who averages between thirty and sixty minutes a day in a variety of activities will burn about 2,000 calories each week. Research shows that activity levels resulting in expenditures of between 1,050 and 2,000 calories a week will decrease the risk of heart disease, in particular.

People who have jobs that are physical—such as carpenters, farmers or waiters—may be getting enough exercise during the workday to expend this number of calories. But they are only a small portion of the American population. Most people need to find extra ways to build more activity into their lives.

Lifetime Physical Activities

Although schools tend to focus on team sports for physical activity, these sports are unlikely to be part of people's lives as they grow older. Most team sports are highly competitive, pitting one person or group against another. While adults may not regularly take part in team sports such as baseball or basketball, they may ski, swim, run or walk.

To be practical in the long term, physical activities taught in school should help to develop lifestyles and skills that can keep people active far into adulthood. These nonteam forms of exercise are called *lifetime physical activities*. Lifetime activities may be readily carried into adulthood because they generally need only one or two people.

Besides activities such as swimming, bicycling and other sports, other vigorous social activities such as dancing are also considered lifetime activities. Many physical educators emphasize the importance of dedicating more curriculum time to lifetime physical activities.

Unfortunately, the mainstays of the school physical education program are still games for younger children and competitive sports for older students. But many physical educators now believe that more emphasis should be given to developing the knowledge, attitudes, cognitive skills and physical skills students need to remain physically active throughout life.

Staying Motivated

People sometimes find it difficult to continue with an exercise program once they have started. The following suggestions help increase motivation.

- **Set realistic goals.** If a plan is too ambitious, it will be hard to maintain. Setting definite goals that are achievable will help.
- **Add variety.** Doing the same kind of activity over and over can become boring. Varying activities helps maintain interest and provides fitness benefits.
- **Record progress.** Before starting, evaluate fitness levels. Record time spent and list achievements.
- **Start slow and easy.** Starting with a ten-minute session three times a week, at moderate intensity, leaves a person feeling good afterward. Workouts can be gradually lengthened and the pace stepped up.
- **Make it convenient.** Time and location should be convenient; otherwise, the lack of convenience will provide a good excuse to stop the activity.
- **Find a support group.** Studies have shown that exercising with a partner helps people stick with an exercise plan and stay motivated.

Ideas for Activity

Exercise activities don't have to be "hard" or repetitious. Variety can help work the various muscle groups. Variety also encourages continued interest in exercise.

Even routine activities that people undertake as part of their normal schedule count in terms of energy expended, or calories burned. One exercise physiologist suggests thinking of calorie-burning in terms of a piggy bank, where every penny counts.

Another way to increase daily activity is to create interruptions. "Mini-walks" can provide breaks throughout the day and can be both physically and mentally refreshing. The idea is to look for opportunities to move—take a short walk, walk up or down stairs, go outside for a few minutes. Fitting mini-walks into the day can provide extra energy and get the body into the habit of small but frequent amounts of activity over the course of a day.

Activities for Fitness

A wide variety of activities can contribute to fitness.

Archery	Table tennis	Ironing
Badminton	Tennis	Mowing lawns
Volleyball	Canoeing	Raking
Croquet	Hiking	Scrubbing floors
Fishing	Water-skiing	Shoveling snow
Golf	Carrying firewood	Climbing stairs
Walking	Chopping wood	Washing cars
Horseback riding	Cooking	Weeding
Racquetball	Digging ditches	Cleaning windows
Scuba diving	Food shopping	Bicycling
Roller-skating	Gardening	Jogging
Ice skating	Hedge trimming	Jumping rope
Cross-country skiing	Soccer	Swimming
Downhill skiing	House cleaning	Weight training

Principles for Improving Fitness

While increasing one's overall activity level can greatly improve long-term health, improving each of the specific elements of fitness offers benefits as well. Once individual levels of fitness have been assessed, improvement in specific elements may be desired. The following general principles can help improve elements of fitness.

- overloading
- specificity
- threshold and target zone
- progression
- frequency, intensity and time (FIT)

■ **Overloading:** To improve fitness, muscles must be "overloaded"—worked against a greater load than normal. A normal amount of exercise maintains the current fitness level. Overloading requires a level of exercise that increases activity above normal (the "threshold" level), but not so high that it causes injury or distress. This area or level of activity is sometimes called the fitness *target zone*. Because individual fitness levels and goals vary, individual target zones will vary, too.

■ **Specificity:** Improving an individual component of fitness requires overloading that is specific to that characteristic. For example, exercises to build muscular strength may not do much to improve cardiorespiratory endurance. Specificity helps to determine appropriate exercises, as well as warm-up and cool-down activities.

■ **Threshold and target zone:** Each component of fitness has a threshold and a target zone. The training threshold is the minimal amount of exercise required for improving fitness. The target zone is the range of activity above normal that is optimal for increasing fitness. Getting too much exercise or going beyond the target zone—for example, by engaging in vigorous activity only on weekends—can result in injury and fail to improve fitness.

As fitness improves, the threshold and target zone may change. They will also change if a person stops exercising for a while. Threshold and target zones are based on the current level of fitness and the current exercise pattern.

- **Progression:** Overload needs to progress at the right pace to be helpful. Beginners should start near the threshold level, where activity is just slightly increased above normal, and make gradual increases in frequency of activity, intensity (or difficulty level) and duration.

- **Frequency, intensity and time (FIT):** For exercise to be effective in improving fitness, it must be done with enough frequency and intensity and for a long enough time. The acronym FIT can be a helpful way to remember these conditions.

  Frequency refers to how often an activity is done. Intensity means that exercise must be hard enough to require more exertion than normal. For example: To increase flexibility, the muscles must be stretched beyond normal length. To increase cardiorespiratory endurance, the heart rate must be increased above its normal pace. To increase strength, the muscles must experience more resistance than normal.

  Time, or duration, of exercise also matters. For improving the individual fitness components, the length of time can be gradually increased.

Ratings for Popular Activities

This chart indicates how some popular activities affect the elements of fitness. A higher number indicates the activity does more to improve an element of fitness; a lower number indicates less effect.

Elements	Jogging	Bicycling	Swimming	Skating	Handball/racquetball	Nordic skiing	Alpine skiing	Basketball	Tennis	Calisthenics	Walking
Aerobic capacity	21	19	21	18	19	19	16	19	16	10	13
Muscular endurance	20	18	20	17	18	19	18	17	16	13	14
Muscular strength	17	16	14	15	15	15	15	15	14	16	11
Flexibility	9	9	15	13	16	14	14	13	14	19	7
Body composition	21	21	15	17	19	17	15	19	16	12	13

Reprinted with permission from B. Hubbard. 1991. *Entering Adulthood: Moving into Fitness*. Santa Cruz, CA: ETR Associates.

Improving Cardiorespiratory Endurance

Many activities can help improve cardiorespiratory endurance, or aerobic fitness. Such activities must place demands on the heart and lungs. Activities should be continuous and involve repetitive movements of the large muscle groups.

Activities that meet this requirement include swimming, bicycling, basketball, cross-country skiing, aerobic dancing, walking and jogging. Activities such as tennis and racquetball can meet the requirement if the action is continuous.

Whichever exercise is chosen, an aerobic workout should follow the same basic pattern:

1. Warm up to elevate body temperature.
2. Stretch to loosen muscles and prevent injury.
3. Exercise at target heart rate.
4. Cool down by moving more slowly.
5. Stretch to prevent muscle soreness.

Frequency

Maintaining or improving cardiorespiratory endurance involves exercising three to six times a week. However, even exercise that is obtained in a piecemeal fashion—such as spending an available five minutes on a stationary bike—is better than no exercise at all.

Intensity

Planned exercise or recreation, such as walking, jogging or cycling, is one way to meet the current recommendation for thirty minutes or more of moderate-intensity physical activity over the course of the day. For those who want to train more seriously, activities should be performed with enough intensity to reach and maintain a *target heart rate* (THR).

The heart rate is used to measure intensity because it is a convenient indicator of oxygen consumption. Cardiorespiratory endurance improves as the muscles' consumption of oxygen and the body's metabolic rate increase. The THR is the number of times the heart needs to beat each minute to have a positive effect on the cardiorespiratory system, also called a *training effect*.

THR is usually calculated at 60% to 90% of the maximum heart rate. Maximum heart rate is usually calculated by subtracting age in years from 220. This formula is based on averages, so it works for most people, but not all. A person whose heart beats unusually fast or slow should use common sense in setting THR, using a pace that is comfortable without feeling excessive fatigue.

The choice of a THR will depend on the current level of fitness. A person who is already in relatively good shape might start exercising at 75% of maximum heart rate. A well-conditioned person may choose an even higher THR. A person with a low initial fitness level can obtain a training effect at a lower THR, such as 60% of maximum heart rate.

Calculating Target Heart Rate

Finding the target heart rate involves subtracting age in years from 220 to get the maximum heart rate, then multiplying by .60 to .90, depending on initial level of fitness. Two examples:

- **For a 15 year old (setting a THR of 80%):**
  Maximum heart rate: 220 – 15 = 205
  205 X .80 = 164 beats per minute

- **For a 40 year old (setting a THR of 60%):**
  Maximum heart rate: 220 – 40 = 180
  180 X .60 = 108 beats per minute

Source: W. A. Payne and D. B. Hahn. 1992. *Understanding Your Health*, 3d ed. St. Louis, MO: Mosby Year Book.

The heart rate can be determined by finding a location on the body where an artery passes near the surface of the skin and then feeling for the pulse. Two good sites are the *carotid artery* (one on either side of the Adam's apple at the front of the throat) and the *radial artery* (on the inside of the wrist, near the base of the thumb).

To find the pulse, the front surface of the index and middle fingertips are placed at one of these locations to feel for a pulse. The thumb should not be used to measure pulse rate, because the thumb has a pulse of its own, which can interfere with pulse counts. Once a regular pulse is felt, the number of beats felt in a six-second period are counted, using a watch or a timer, and then multiplied by ten.

Tips for Beginning Exercisers

1. **If you can't do it right, do it often.** Don't be too rigid in adhering to the "rules" about aerobic exercise. If necessary, quantity can take the place of quality.
2. **Don't exercise with a fit friend**—unless the pace is adjusted to meet the needs of a beginner. To avoid getting injured, don't push yourself beyond your fitness level.
3. **Start so slowly that people make fun of you.** By starting off at a slow pace—such as at 65% of your maximum heart rate—your body will adapt to and benefit from the exercise.
4. **Exercise as often as possible.** The more activity a person does, the greater the improvement in fitness.

Source: C. Bailey. 1991. *The New Fit or Fat.* Boston: Houghton Mifflin.

Time

At least 25 minutes of continuous aerobic activity two or three times a week are required to produce a training effect. Generally, the duration can be shorter for people using a high intensity form of exercise. Those using activities with a lower range of intensity should maintain the activity for a longer time.

Improving Body Composition

Body composition can be improved by making good nutrition and regular exercise a part of the normal routine. Particularly helpful are reducing dietary fat (especially saturated fat) to minimal levels and getting moderate exercise every day to increase caloric expenditure and maintain muscle tone, joint flexibility and bone strength. It is important to be realistic about what can and cannot be changed, and to remember—despite the many social pressures to the contrary—that diversity in body size and shape is normal.

Body composition differs from the other components of fitness in that specific areas of the body cannot be changed through diet or exercise. Spot reduction—doing sit-ups to try to reduce abdominal fat or leg raises to reduce fat in the thighs—does not work. These exercises may build underlying muscle tissue, but the fatty tissue will remain.

The exercise that can work to change body composition is systemic, or aerobic, exercise. For example, bicycling or jogging will have the effect of reducing body fat overall. Body fat located in the abdominal area, which poses the greatest health risk, is more easily lost than fat located elsewhere in the body. Fat in the hips and thighs is more resistant to weight loss.

The Role of Good Nutrition

Good nutritional habits that can help to improve body composition include:

- limiting fat in the diet
- increasing consumption of complex carbohydrates
- avoiding fad diets
- eating a variety of healthy foods

■ **Limiting fat in the diet:** Probably the most significant dietary change that can lead to improvements in body composition is a reduction in dietary fat, especially saturated fat.

Not all fat is bad for health. Some fat in the diet is necessary. Fat helps distribute and store the fat-soluble vitamins A, D, E and K; it keeps skin adequately lubricated; and it contributes to the production of *prostaglandins*, which control many important body processes.

However, the amount of fat needed to perform these functions is less than one-twelfth of the amount most Americans now consume. A diet with only 3% of calories from fat would be enough to carry out fat's vital functions, but the average American gets about 40% of calories from fat.

The type of fat needed by the body is *unsaturated fat.* Although the body does not require *saturated fat,* most Americans consume much more saturated than unsaturated fat. Saturated fat occurs primarily in animal foods—meats, eggs, milk, butter and cheese. A diet high in saturated fat can cause the liver to increase its output of cholesterol, especially *low-density lipoprotein* (LDL) cholesterol—the harmful type that clogs arteries.

LDL cholesterol is not a fuel and can't be burned through exercise. Only diet can control LDL cholesterol. Exercise can boost HDL cholesterol—the "good" kind of cholesterol that helps protect against heart disease—but fairly rigorous exercise over a long period of time is required for this effect. Keeping LDL levels low through a healthy diet can reduce the body's need for high levels of HDL.

Because dietary fat is similar to body fat, it requires very little biochemical energy to become body fat. The body can convert calories from dietary fat into body fat more efficiently than it can calories from carbohydrates. Therefore, an individual can lose weight, including body fat, by switching to a diet low in fats and high in complex carbohydrates—even if the number of calories consumed stays the same.

The body naturally tries to avoid turning carbohydrates into fat. To burn off extra calories from carbohydrates, the body increases its metabolic rate. Also, the thermic effect of food—the energy cost associated with digestion and absorption—is higher for carbohydrates. Walking immediately after eating raises this effect even higher.

For all of these reasons, a diet high in fat is much more apt to put on weight and increase the percentage of body fat than a diet equal in calories but lower in fat. This is true of all types of fat, not just saturated fat. All fats contain nine calories per gram—so reducing total dietary fat is the way to reduce fat accumulation in the body. The fats that are consumed should be primarily of the polyunsaturated or monounsaturated variety.

The American Heart Association recommends that no more than 30% of calories in the diet come from fat. However, many authorities call for even less—about 20%.

- **Increasing consumption of complex carbohydrates:** Many people think of complex carbohydrates, or starches, as fattening. However, this idea is totally unfounded. Dietary starches are the best fuel for muscular as well as mental energy. They keep the body steadily supplied with blood sugar, the only fuel that can be used by the brain.

  Complex carbohydrates include whole-grain cereals and breads, brown rice, potatoes, beans, pastas, fruits and vegetables. Some experts suggest getting 65% of calories from complex carbohydrates. These foods should be rich in vital nutrients—foods with high *nutrient density*. Such foods offer good nutritional value in relationship to their caloric value.

HEALTHY CARBOHYDRATE CHOICES

- Choose whole-grain or 100% whole-wheat breads.
- Bake or boil potatoes, and go easy on additions that contain fat.
- Eat lots of pasta—but beware of high-fat sauces (such as the creamy, cheesy types).
- Enjoy low-calorie snacks, such as raw vegetables, popcorn (skip the butter and salt) and pretzels.

■ **Avoiding fad diets:** Fad diets can actually result in the development of more, not less, body fat. Yo-yo dieting (losing, then gaining weight) is a pattern that can result in added fat, and research shows that it also can increase risks to health.

Fasting is one type of diet that can encourage the body to become fatter. When the body is deprived of food, it becomes stressed and tries to lay down extra fat for the emergency. Eating just one meal a day can also have this effect. This response is a "safety device" that developed as an adaptation to protect against famine. Diets that are high in protein and low in carbohydrate trigger the same effect.

■ **Eating a variety of foods from the basic food groups:** Food groups are simply ways of grouping foods of similar nutrient content to help in planning for good nutrition. The U.S. Department of Agriculture has designed a food grouping system, the Food Guide Pyramid, that emphasizes the value of obtaining most energy intake from carbohydrates while limiting fat intake.

The six food groupings are shown as a pyramid, depicting the relative quantities of foods that should be consumed in a balanced diet. Foods at the broad base of the pyramid—breads, cereals, rice and pasta—should form the largest part of the diet. Those in the middle of the pyramid—vegetables, fruits, dairy and other protein sources—should be eaten in moderate amounts. Foods at the top—fats, oils and sweets—should be eaten sparingly.

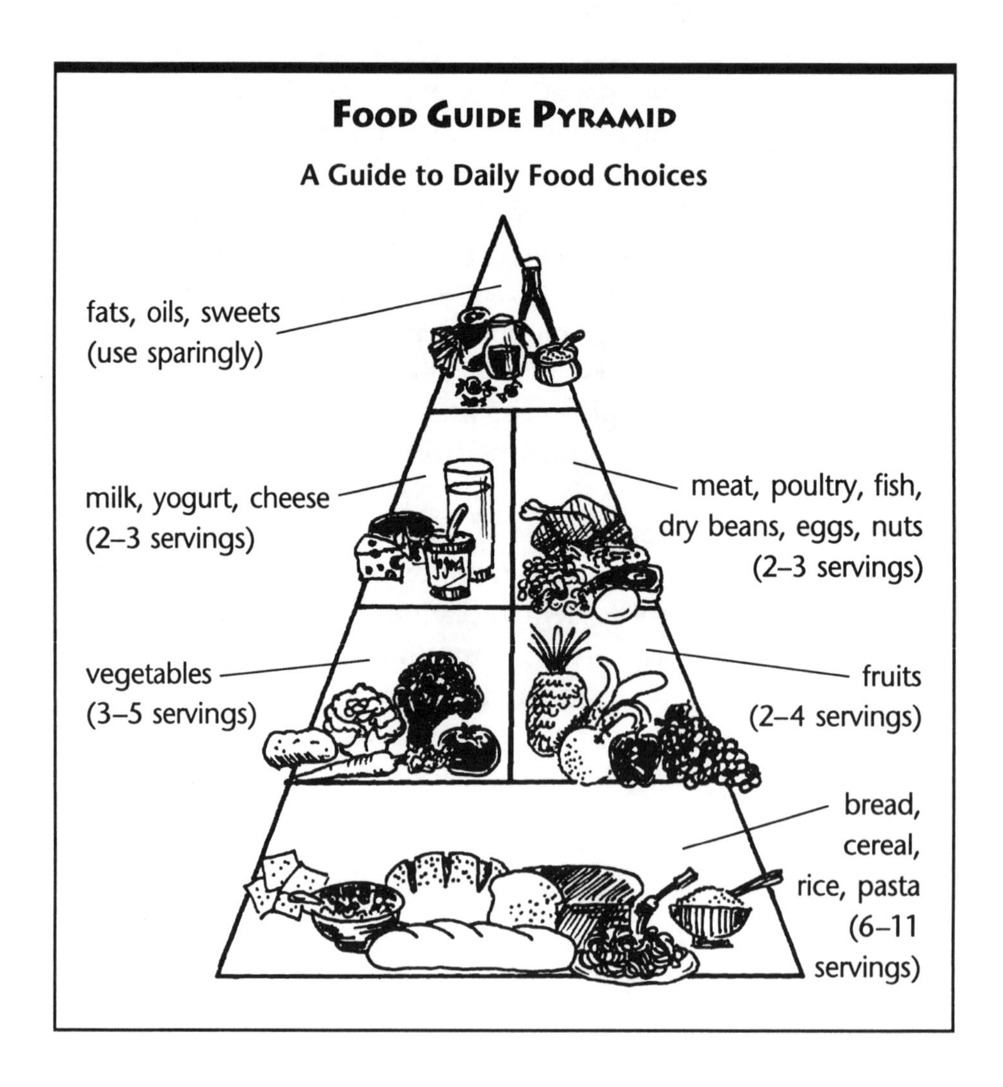

Improving Flexibility

A person becomes more flexible by making stretching part of her or his daily activity. Stretching has the following benefits:

- It helps prevent injuries such as muscle strains and shin splints.
- It reduces muscle tension and induces relaxation.
- It serves as a warm-up for vigorous physical activities.

Static or *sustained stretching* is the safest way to stretch. In a static stretch, a muscle is slowly stretched and then held in the stretched position for several seconds. Static stretching is done to reduce the danger of tearing the soft tissue.

When stretching, a person should reach to the point of discomfort, then back off slightly. The goal is to relax and hold the stretch for ten to twenty seconds. The stretch should never be painful.

Guidelines for Safe Stretching

- Before stretching, increase body temperature by running in place slowly or doing some other rhythmic activity. Raising the body temperature increases flexibility and reduces the risk of injury.
- Breathe slowly and rhythmically throughout the stretches.
- Perform each stretch regularly. If stretching is not done regularly, flexibility is lost.
- Don't do any stretches that involve deep knee bends or full squats. These activities can injure the knees and lower back.

Improving Muscular Strength and Endurance

Muscular strength and endurance can be improved by demanding more work from the muscles, or overloading them. It is important not to quit exercising when the muscles start to tire.

Muscle training is very specific. To build up the arms, one must overload the arm muscles. Overloading the leg muscles will not increase muscular strength anywhere else.

Reps and *sets* are the building blocks of the workout. Reps are repetitions of an exercise. To do a sit-up for eight reps means to perform it eight times in a row before resting. A set is one group of reps followed by a rest interval. Performing eight sit-ups, resting 45 seconds to a minute, then doing eight more sit-ups equals two sets.

A workout for muscular strength or endurance should include eight to twelve reps of each exercise for three sets. When an exercise becomes easy to do, weight can be added to the barbells, dumbbells or other equipment.

Popular methods of improving muscular strength and endurance include:

- exercising with free weights (hand-held weights, dumbbells and barbells)
- using exercise machines (Universal, Hydrofitness, Nautilus, Taurus and Avita)
- doing calisthenics (sit-ups, push-ups, leg raises and others)

Improving muscular strength has different requirements than improving muscular endurance. To increase strength, a few repetitions (usually five to eight) are done with heavy loads. To improve muscular endurance, more repetitions (usually ten to fourteen) are done with lighter loads.

Guidelines for Improving Strength and Endurance

- Have an exercise instructor demonstrate the proper use of the equipment if free weights or machines are being used.
- Don't exercise alone. Use a spotter if barbells are being used.
- Warm up and stretch before beginning.
- Exhale when lifting and inhale when releasing.
- Gradually increase the level of exercise.
- Allow at least 48 hours for muscles to recover from a workout. Workouts on consecutive days may do more harm than good, because the body cannot adapt that quickly.
- Don't let more than four days pass without working out. Muscles will begin to break down if more than three or four days pass without exercising.

1-Minute Facts

- Moderate increases in daily activity level can improve health.

- Physical activities taught in school should help develop lifetime physical activities, lifestyles and skills that can keep people active into adulthood.

- Even routine activities that people undertake as part of their normal schedule can help improve fitness.

- The following general principles can help improve elements of fitness: overloading; specificity; threshold and target zone; progression; and frequency, intensity and time.

- Activities to improve aerobic fitness should be continuous and should involve repetitive movements of the large muscle groups.

- Body composition can be improved by making good nutrition and regular exercise part of the normal routine.

- Stretching increases flexibility.

- Muscular strength and endurance can be improved by demanding more work from the muscles, or overloading them.

PREPARING FOR FITNESS

MYTH: You really have to be an exercise fanatic to discipline yourself enough to get regular exercise.

Fact: Getting regular exercise requires planning and fitting appropriate exercise and activities into a daily schedule. Exercise can become a healthy habit when people choose to make it part of their daily routine.

According to one survey, people who exercise regularly fit their workouts into their existing daily schedule, rather than adding special time for exercise. Ways to fit exercise into daily routine include:

- Walk or bike to school or work.
- Substitute an active for an inactive pastime, e.g., playing sports instead of video games after school.
- Take the stairs instead of using elevators or escalators.

The time of day a person exercises can affect the activities that follow. Fitness experts suggest planning to work out just before doing activities that require the greatest concentration.

Workouts should be scheduled at least two hours before planning to go to sleep. Vigorous exercise just before bedtime can interfere with sleep.

Exercise can be planned for indoors or outdoors. When exercising outdoors, isolated places should be avoided for safety reasons. Security can be increased by taking friends along, which can also make an activity more enjoyable.

Some important considerations in planning to increase physical fitness include:

- reducing the risk of injury
- preparing for the weather
- having comfortable and safe clothing and equipment
- taking good care of the feet
- meeting fluid and nutrient needs
- getting adequate sleep and rest

Reducing the Risk of Injury

While the risk of injury cannot be eliminated altogether, it can be reduced. Exercise plans should be based on the specific needs of the individual, including the current level of fitness and any known health limitations. Someone who has a condition such as asthma or knee problems should discuss the condition with a doctor before beginning an exercise program. Programs often can be modified to accommodate the limitations.

The following basic rules help prevent injury.

■ **Always warm up and cool down.** Warming up prepares the body for exercise by gradually increasing the heart rate and blood flow, raising the temperature of muscles and connective tissue and improving muscle function. A warm-up period should precede stretching, as stretching cold muscles can injure them. Warming up can be general, such as jogging in place, or it can be specific, such as doing a less vigorous version of the exercise that will follow.

Cooling down not only reduces muscle stiffness but also can prevent an abrupt drop in blood pressure that occurs when vigorous activity is suddenly stopped. Exercisers should never stand still immediately after vigorous exercise.

In cold weather, exercisers should warm up before going outdoors, and cool down indoors as well. Many exercisers find that in cold weather, they can stretch more fully indoors.

- **Don't overdo it.** Any new exercise should be begun at a lower level of intensity and the level of exertion increased gradually over several weeks. Studies show that the most common cause of injury is doing too much, too soon.

- **Stop if pain is felt while exercising.** Pain felt during exercise may indicate a problem. Muscle soreness that develops after exercise usually means that there was insufficient warming up or that the muscles are being worked too long or too hard. Sore muscles do not mean a person should stop exercising, but that he or she should slow down.

- **Use controlled movements.** Rapid, jerky movement can lead to injury. As the limbs are moved, the muscles should be kept contracted and should be moved as if pushing against some resistance.

- **Don't bounce while stretching.** Bouncing movements can actually shorten muscles and increase the chance of muscle tears and soreness. "Static" or gradual stretches loosen muscles without straining them.

- **Avoid high-impact aerobics.** High-impact aerobics can cause injury to shins, calves, ankles, knees and the lower back. Low-impact aerobics can easily raise the heart rate enough to provide health benefits.

Preparing for the Weather

Temperature and humidity should be considered when planning to exercise. Exercising in extremes of weather can be exhilarating, whether hiking in the summer heat or walking in the snow. But good judgment is needed, along with awareness of potential hazards associated with weather conditions. A combination of taking a few simple precautions and having the right gear can help prevent injury.

Wearing light colors and fabrics in hot weather allows the body to dissipate heat. Rubberized or plastic clothing should never be worn. During the first few hot days of the season, take it easy to allow the body to adjust to the warmer weather. Someone who feels weak and tired while exercising should stop and drink several ounces of water.

In cold weather, layers of loose-fitting, thin clothing, which can be removed as the body warms up, are most comfortable. Thermal underwear made of a fabric that draws sweat away from the skin (such as polypropylene, Capilene or Thermax) is a good first layer. Cotton holds moisture next to the skin, causing a person to become cold and clammy. A wool sweater or a synthetic turtleneck works well for the middle layer. Sweat pants, lycra tights or leg warmers will help keep legs warm; they can be worn over thermal long johns during very cold weather. A light jacket that is waterproof and wind resistant yet breathable (such as Gore-Tex) is best for the outer layer.

Since about 40% of body heat is lost through the head and neck, wearing a cap or other head covering is important for staying warm. The areas most sensitive to cold are fingers, toes and ears. Protecting these with mittens, wool socks and a cap reduces the discomfort and danger of exposure to low temperatures.

Snow-covered ground can reflect the sun and burn the face, as well as obscure vision. Wearing sunglasses and sunscreen can prevent these problems. Sunglasses and sunscreen should be worn during all daytime outdoor activity.

Clothing and Equipment

Appropriate clothing and equipment are important for both comfort and safety. For most activities, clothing should be light and loose-fitting. In warm weather, cotton shorts and T-shirts are a good choice. For outside activity in cold weather, the essentials include a hat that covers the ears, mittens and several thin layers of clothing that can be peeled off when the exerciser warms up.

Equipment should be appropriate for the activity. For example, protective padding for knees and elbows should be worn when skateboarding or roller-skating. A helmet should always be worn when riding a bicycle. The safest helmets are fully enclosed on top with a foam liner inside to absorb the impact of a fall. Since the plastics used in helmets deteriorate with weather and wear, helmets should be replaced every five years.

For cycling at night, a headlight and taillight should be used. Reflective clothing and patches help create visibility for cyclists as well as walkers and runners. The most visible way to wear a reflective stripe is horizontally, across the full width of the back. Wearing light clothing at night is not enough. A person dressed all in white is visible at a distance of only a little more than two hundred feet, usually not enough space for a driver to swerve or stop.

Caring for the Feet

Taking good care of the feet is critical. Many specialized athletic shoes are on the market now, and the variety can be confusing. But the proper shoe for the activity can make a big difference in terms of performance, health and enjoyment.

Athletic Shoes and Socks

Athletic shoes are built from two basic types: running shoes and tennis-type or court shoes. Running shoes are good for activities that involve mostly forward movement. These shoes are light-weight with deeply cut tread, a thick heel wedge that tilts the body forward and a breathable upper.

Court shoes are best for activities that involve mostly side-to-side movement, including all racquet sports. They are heavier and stiffer than running shoes, with flat soles. Aerobics shoes combine the features of running and court shoes. Court shoes can be used in aerobics classes; running shoes should not be. Walking shoes should have rubber heels; they may also have curved soles to facilitate the rocking motion of walking.

Tips For Selecting the Right Shoes

Running Shoes:

- Check the wear pattern on the shoes being replaced. If soles are worn on both inside and outside edges, support is more important than cushioning. If soles are worn predominantly on the outside edges, support can be sacrificed for cushioning.
- Know whether feet are curved or straight and whether arches are high or flat. The shoe should fit the shape of the foot.
- Find a knowledgeable salesperson who can provide advice.

Court Shoes:

- For tennis, look for side support and soles with good traction.
- For racquetball, choose side support over flexibility and cushioning.

Aerobics Shoes:

- Check the width of the shoe at the widest part of the foot. The bottom of the shoe should be as wide as the bottom of the foot, and the uppers shouldn't go over the sides.
- Choose leather or nylon uppers. Leather is more durable, but it can stretch.

Socks have also been designed for specific sports, such as tennis, cycling, running, skiing and aerobics. They differ according to where protective padding is located, how thick the padding is and what materials are used. But while sports-specific socks can help avoid foot abrasion, the sock is not as important as the appropriate shoe.

Some Common Foot Problems

Common foot problems that may interfere with exercising and require attention include:

- athlete's foot
- ingrown toenails
- blisters
- corns and calluses
- bunions

■ **Athlete's foot** can be avoided by keeping feet clean and dry. Athlete's foot is caused by a fungus that thrives in warm, moist environments—not only locker rooms or gym showers. Poorly ventilated shoes and damp, sweaty socks are ideal breeding grounds.

Athlete's foot is characterized by itching toes, soles or sides of the feet, along with tiny blisters and sometimes red scaling in these areas and between the toes. Usually, the fungus can be effectively treated with an over-the-counter antifungal preparation. If the condition does not clear up in a week or two, or if the area becomes red and swollen, medical attention should be sought.

To avoid athlete's foot, the feet should be kept clean and dry. Going barefoot as much as possible can help. Socks that "wick" away moisture and keep the feet dry should be worn.

- **Ingrown toenails** may be the most common of all foot afflictions. They usually occur on the big toe, where they cause swelling and redness and can lead to infection. There are two causes: tight shoes or stockings that press the nail into the tissue, and improper trimming of the toenail.

  To avoid ingrown toenails, nails should be cut straight across, with the edge of the nail a square, not a half moon. Nails should not be trimmed too close. If an ingrown toenail develops, the cause should be determined and avoided. The toe can be soaked in warm water and a few strands of absorbent cotton pressed under the nail to keep it from cutting the skin. If possible, open-toed shoes should be worn while the toe heals. If pus, bleeding or painful swelling occurs, medical advice should be obtained.

- **Blisters** are abrasion injuries, which can be caused by ill-fitting shoes, socks or stockings. Shoes that usually fit well can cause blisters if socks or stockings are not worn, especially in hot weather.

  Small blisters usually heal by themselves. They should be kept clean and covered with a thin foam pad or light bandage. If there are any signs of infection, a doctor should be seen.

- **Corns and calluses** are the skin's response to pressure and chafing. People with flat feet are more susceptible to them. Corns usually appear on or between the toes, calluses under the heel or on the ball of the foot.

  The size of both corns and calluses can be reduced by soaking the foot in warm water until the hardened skin softens, then gently rubbing the skin with a pumice stone. A light bandage or adhesive-backed moleskin can be used after treatments. The cause should be determined so that other choices in footwear can be made. In severe cases, corns and calluses may require medical treatment to remove them.

- **Bunions** are bony outgrowths that develop at the big toe joint. They are both disfiguring and painful. If they are neglected over a long period of time, they can seriously interfere with walking and standing. The tendency to develop bunions may be hereditary, and flat-footed people are more likely to get them than others. Poor-fitting shoes, especially those with high heels and narrow toes, are considered the worst bunion-makers. For this reason, women are more prone to bunions than men.

  If a bunion is developing, a person should switch to shoes with a low heel and ample room in the toe. Soaking feet in warm water at night and gentle massage may also relieve pain. In severe cases, bunions may require surgical removal.

IN OTHER PARTS OF THE WORLD...

About one billion people worldwide wear no shoes at all. The few surveys that have been done on barefoot populations have shown that they seem to have fewer foot problems.

Meeting Fluid and Nutrient Needs

The body loses fluid through sweating, even in cool temperatures. However, the need for fluid during physical activity does not always cause a feeling of thirst. Exercisers need to make a conscious effort to drink enough fluids when exercising.

In hot weather, a person can easily lose more than a quart of water an hour through sweating. During endurance activities such as long-distance cycling, marathon running or cross-country skiing, the effects can be severe, and heat exhaustion or heat stroke can occur. Research shows that cool drinks are absorbed more quickly than lukewarm ones.

Water is the ideal fluid replacement, because it is absorbed more efficiently than any other beverage. Specially formulated sports drinks may not have any more benefits than water unless they are being used for long workouts (two hours or more). In addition, sports drinks can cause nausea in some people.

Sugary drinks, including soft drinks, should be avoided before exercising. These drinks can decrease endurance, due to the body's production of insulin in response to the sugar. Beverages containing caffeine (colas, teas and coffee) should be avoided, because they stimulate fluid loss in the body. Alcohol also should be avoided, because it hinders coordination and impairs performance. Alcohol also promotes the loss of fluid from the body.

Salt lost through sweating does not need to be replaced with additional salt or salt tablets. Americans consume enough salt in their diet to replace the salt lost in sweating. Salt tablets can lead to dehydration and elevated blood pressure, and should not be used.

For most people who exercise to improve fitness, eating a balanced diet supplies the body with the necessary nutrients. In some endurance sports such as marathon running, athletes find that carbohydrate loading ("carbo loading") increases the energy source, glycogen, in their muscles. But the improvement in performance, if any, is usually small. A balanced daily diet should be high in complex carbohydrates.

For less strenuous levels of physical activity, the body's fuel comes from foods eaten hours or even days earlier. Therefore, eating a candy bar or other food high in sugar before exercising does not provide the sustained energy that is needed.

People who eat a balanced diet do not need to take vitamin, mineral or other supplements (such as protein powders). Excessive amounts of vitamins and minerals can be dangerous, and supplements do not provide the combination of nutrients that are supplied by eating a variety of foods.

Sleep and Rest

Sleep is an indispensable part of a fitness program. During sleep, people recover from physical and emotional stresses and injuries. An added benefit of exercise is that it is often associated with improvements in sleeping. However, exercising just before bedtime can interfere with sleep.

Sleep needs vary depending on activity level, overall health and age. Young people generally require about eight to ten hours of sleep each night. Growth hormone is secreted almost exclusively during sleep—and growth hormone provides for the growth and repair of body cells.

A good night's sleep is mentally and physiologically rejuvenating. When a person is low on sleep, all body systems work less efficiently. Lack of sleep causes irritability, loss of coordination and difficulty concentrating.

Special Concerns

Some specific concerns have arisen in terms of both behavior and physiology related to sports and efforts to improve fitness. These include:

- the use of *anabolic steroids* for muscular growth and weight gain
- the development of menstrual irregularity, or *amenorrhea*, in some female athletes
- the issue of gender equity in school sports

■ **Anabolic steroids** are synthetic drugs that simulate the male hormone *testosterone*. Steroids can be taken in tablet form or by injection. They are used medically to treat certain diseases. In small doses, they can be helpful in treating or repairing soft tissue injuries, skeletal disorders, malnutrition and some forms of anemia.

Some athletes and bodybuilders have used steroids to stimulate muscle growth and weight gain. While steroids promote increased strength and bulk, the health risks outweigh any benefit. Steroid use can result in liver damage, infertility, kidney disorders, hardening of the arteries and mental disorders such as severe depression, aggression and violence and extreme moodiness. The abuse of steroids can lead to death.

It is estimated that more than a million people in the United States use or have used anabolic steroids. About half of this group are adolescents, who face serious potential health problems as a result. For this group, growth can be halted when the steroids seal off bone development. Steroids are psychologically and physiologically addictive.

Men who take steroids may experience breast growth, reduced sperm production and shrinking of the testicles. Side effects for women include growth of facial and body hair, baldness, a lowering of the voice, decreased breast size, menstrual irregularities and enlarged genitals. People who inject steroids may be exposed to HIV, the virus that causes AIDS, if they share needles. Long-term use may lead to heart disease and other cardiovascular disease.

- **Amenorrhea** is the temporary absence of menstruation. Amenorrhea has been observed in women who participate in strenuous physical activities, including distance running, ballet dancing and weight lifting. The exact cause of the cessation of menstruation during times of intensive training is not known. About 20% of female athletes and only 5% of other women experience amenorrhea.

  One hypothesis is that intensive running and similar activities reduce body weight and put women below a body fat threshold necessary for menstruation. However, exercise is not the only possible cause of amenorrhea. Irregular periods may also be caused by serious medical conditions, such as a pituitary gland tumor or an underactive thyroid. Amenorrhea can also be caused by emotional stress and dieting. A doctor should be consulted to determine the cause of amenorrhea.

  Amenorrhea in athletes is not permanent and does not indicate sterility. In general, amenorrhea occurs in young, competitive women who train intensely, not in women who exercise for fitness.

- **Gender equity in school sports** is a concern in many communities. Despite the passage in 1972 of Title IX—a law that guarantees equal opportunity for males and females in all aspects of education, including sports—opportunities and participation in high school and college sports remain unequal for men and women. The law covers most aspects of high school and college sports, including scholarships, budgets, participation, coaches' salaries and gender, equipment and facilities.

  Since the federal law was passed, gains have been made in some areas. The total number of girls participating in high school sports has increased by 10% since 1981. (The number of boys increased by less than 1%.) However, almost twice as many boys as girls participate in high school sports.

At the college level, although more than 50% of students are women, a much smaller proportion participates in sports. A national study of 250 colleges found that almost 70% of scholarship funds and almost 83% of recruiting funds were spent on men. Male students received more than three-quarters of team operating funds. While the student bodies were just over 50% female, only about 30% of all participants in athletics were female.

Part of the problem seems to be that often those in charge of implementing the law do not fully understand it. But there are other factors at work, too. For example, in one college the number of women coaching women's sports dwindled from 90% when Title IX took effect to only 30% in 1992. The decrease was an unforeseen result of the fact that the law raised salaries for women's coaches and administrators, prompting more men to apply for those jobs.

For many schools, complaints to the national Office of Civil Rights have been necessary to initiate the transition to gender equity. In some states, legal action has been initiated to bring high schools and colleges into compliance with Title IX. As a result, by the 1998/99 school year, each campus with an NCAA (National Collegiate Athletic Association) program must meet specific guidelines for gender equity in sports activities.

Athletics, like other physical fitness activities, do not have gender boundaries. Both men and women benefit from physical activity.

1-Minute Facts

- Getting regular exercise requires planning.
- Planning exercise based on the specific needs of the individual and following basic safety rules can help prevent injury during exercise.
- Temperature and humidity should be considered when planning to exercise.
- Appropriate clothing and equipment are important for both comfort and safety.
- Proper care of the feet, including the right kind of shoes, can help prevent foot problems and injury.
- Exercisers need to make a conscious effort to drink plenty of fluids during exercise.
- Sleep is an indispensable part of a fitness program.
- Specific concerns around exercise include the use of steroids, menstrual irregularities and gender equity in school sports.

Glossary

A

aerobic—The form of energy production in the body that requires the presence of oxygen; it is used for activities such as walking or jogging.

aerobic fitness—See cardiorespiratory endurance.

amenorrhea—The temporary absence of menstruation.

anabolic steroids—Synthetic drugs that stimulate the production of the male hormone testosterone.

anaerobic—The oxygen-deprived form of energy production; it is used for activities such as weight lifting or sprinting.

B

basal metabolic rate—The rate at which calories are used to sustain life functions during rest.

body composition—The proportion of body fat to lean tissue in an individual, usually given as the percentage of body weight that is fat.

C

carbohydrate loading ("carbo loading")—Ingestion of foods high in carbohydrates (preferably complex) prior to endurance sports or intensive training to improve performance.

cardiorespiratory endurance—The body's ability to take in and use oxygen so that muscles can function; its level is dependent on cardiorespiratory capacity and the ability of cells in the body to efficiently use oxygen and release carbon dioxide. Also known as aerobic fitness.

cardiovascular—Of, relating to or involving the heart and blood vessels.

E

ectomorph—A body type that is tall and thin.

endomorph—A body type that is short and rounded.

endorphin—Any of several chemicals produced by the brain that help relieve pain.

F

FIT—An acronym helpful for remembering the relationship between the components of Frequency, Intensity and Time when using exercise to improve fitness.

fitness—A combination of qualities that enable an individual to meet the physical demands of life.

flexibility—The elasticity of muscles and connective tissues, which determines the range of motion of the joints.

H

HDL (high-density lipoprotein)—A type of lipoprotein that carries cholesterol from the bloodstream to the liver, where it can be excreted from the body. HDL may protect individuals against coronary artery disease.

heredity—Inheritance of qualities and potentials of one's ancestors.

hydrostatic weighing—A method for determining body composition.

L

lactic acid—A byproduct of anaerobic respiration that can cause discomfort by increasing the acidity in the body.

LDL (low-density lipoprotein)—A type of lipoprotein that carries cholesterol from the digestive tract to other body tissues; implicated in the accumulation of plaque within arteries.

lifetime physical activities—Nonteam physical activities that can be used throughout life for the purpose of improving or maintaining physical fitness.

mesomorph—A muscular body type.

muscular endurance—The ability of muscle tissue to persist in an activity.

muscular strength—The force that muscles can exert upon contraction for the purpose of bodily movement and support.

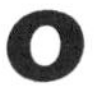

obesity—A condition in which an abnormal proportion of body tissue is fat.

overloading—Increasing the work done by muscles to above normal levels, but below the loads that would cause injury or distress, to improve fitness.

oxygen debt—When the oxygen demands of the muscles cannot be met during physical activity; makes an activity anaerobic.

P

prostaglandin—Any of a group of hormonelike substances found throughout the body that control important body processes.

S

skinfold measurements—A simple method of measuring body composition, which uses calipers to measure the thickness of folds of skin.

T

target heart rate (THR)—A figure used to determine the number of heartbeats per minute required to positively affect the cardiorespiratory system during exercise.

target zone—The range of above-normal activity that optimizes an increase in fitness.

thermic effect of food—A physiological phenomenon characterized by an increase of the body's metabolic rate by about 10% due to the processes of digestion.

training threshold—The minimal amount of exercise that is required to improve fitness.

V

VO_2 max—A laboratory test called the maximal oxygen consumption. It is used to measure aerobic fitness, the results being expressed as the amount of oxygen consumed per body weight.

Resources

Aerobics and Fitness Association of America
15250 Ventura Blvd., Suite 200
Sherman Oaks, CA 91403
800-233-4886

American Alliance for Health, Physical Education, Recreation and Dance
1900 Association Dr.
Reston, VA 22091
703-476-3400
Publications office: 800-321-0789

American Council on Exercise
5820 Oberlin Dr., Suite 102
San Diego, CA 92121
619-535-8227

Centers for Disease Control and Prevention (CDC)
1600 Clinton Rd. NE
Atlanta, GA 30333
404-639-3311

National Heart, Lung and Blood Institute
Education Programs Information Center
P.O. Box 30105
Bethesda, MD 20824
301-251-1222

National Wellness Association
1045 Clark St., Suite 210
Stevens Point, WI 54481
715-342-2969
fax: 715-342-2979

President's Council on Physical Fitness and Sports
701 Pennsylvania Ave. NW, Room 250
Washington, DC 20004
202-272-3430

United States Olympic Committee
1 Olympic Plaza
Colorado Springs, CO 80909
719-632-5551

Women's Sports Foundation
Eisenhower Park
East Meadow, NY 11554
800-227-3988

YMCA of the USA
101 N. Wacker Dr.
Chicago, IL 60606
800-872-9622

References

Alvarado, D. 1990. In shape in a hurry. *San Jose Mercury News,* 9 May.

Apodaca, J. 1992. *Physical fitness.* In *World book encyclopedia,* vol. 15, 436-437. Chicago: World Book.

Berryman, J., and K. Breighner. 1994. *Modeling healthy behavior.* Santa Cruz, CA: ETR Associates.

Blair, S., H. Kohl III, R. Paffenbarger, Jr., et al. 1989. Physical fitness and all-cause mortality. *Journal of the American Medical Association* 262 (17): 2395-2401.

Brody, J. 1982. *Jane Brody's The New York Times guide to personal health.* New York: Times Books.

Consumer Guide. 1988. Walking for health and fitness. *Consumer Guide Magazine Health Series,* vol. 491, November.

Corbin, C., and R. Lindsey. 1988. *Concepts of physical fitness with laboratories.* Dubuque, IA: Wm. C. Brown.

Farquhar, J. 1987. *The American way of life need not be hazardous to your health.* Reading, MA: Addison-Wesley.

Garzino, M. 1991. *Into adolescence: Fitness, health and hygiene.* Santa Cruz, CA: ETR Associates.

Getchell, L., G. Pippin and J. Varnes. 1994. *Perspectives on health.* Lexington, MA: D.C. Heath and Company.

Glover, B., and J. Shepherd. 1989. *The family fitness handbook.* New York: Penguin Books.

Gottlieb, W., and M. Bricklin, eds. 1984. *Fitness for everyone.* Emmaus, PA: Rodale Press.

Green, L. 1990. *Community health.* St. Louis, MO: Times Mirror/Mosby College Publishing.

Health Education Reports 15 (16): 3-5. August 12, 1993.

Hubbard, B. 1991. *Entering adulthood: Moving into fitness.* Santa Cruz, CA: ETR Associates.

Ikeda, J., and P. Naworski. 1992. *Am I fat? Helping young children accept differences in body size.* Santa Cruz, CA: ETR Associates.

Macmillan health encyclopedia: Nutrition and fitness. 1989. New York: Macmillan.

Mee, C., Jr., ed. 1987. *The fit body: Building endurance.* Alexandria, VA: Time-Life Books.

Mendoza, M. 1993. Title IX: A level playing field? *Santa Cruz Sentinel,* 3 October.

Nelson, H., and R. Jermain. 1991. *Introduction to physical anthropology,* 5th ed. St. Paul, MN: West Publishing.

Ornstein, R., and D. Sobel. 1989. *Healthy pleasures.* Reading, MA: Addison-Wesley.

Papenfuss, R. Physical fitness: A vital component for total health and high-level wellness. In *The comprehensive school health challenge,* vol. 1, ed. P. Cortese and K. Middleton, 491-521. Santa Cruz, CA: ETR Associates.

Pate, R. R. 1988. The evolving definition of physical fitness. *Quest* 40: 174-179.

Pate, R. R. 1990. Health and fitness through physical education: Research directions for the 1990s. In *New possibilities, new paradigms? American Academy of Physical Education Papers No. 24,* 62-69. Champaign, IL: Human Kinetics.

Pate, R. R. 1991. Health-related measures of children's physical fitness. *Journal of School Health* 61 (5): 231-233.

Pate, R. R. 1993. Physical activity in children and youth: Relationship to obesity. *Contemporary Nutrition* 18 (2).

Pate, R. R., M. Dowda and J. G. Ross. 1990. Associations between physical activity and physical fitness in American children. *American Journal of Diseases of Children* 144: 1123-1129.

Pate, R. R., and D. S. Ward. 1990. Endurance exercise trainability in children and youth. *Advances in Sports Medicine and Fitness*, vol. 3. Chicago: Yearbook Medical Publishers.

Payne, W. A., and D. B. Hahn. 1992. *Understanding your health*, 3d ed. St. Louis, MO: Mosby Year Book.

Peterson, A. 1993. Gender equity suit is settled. *Santa Cruz Sentinel*, 23 October.

Sagan, L. 1987. *The health of nations*. New York: Basic Books.

Samuels, M., and N. Samuels. 1988. *The well adult*. New York: Simon and Schuster.

Sharkey, B. 1990. *Physiology of fitness*. Champaign, IL: Human Kinetics.

Stamford, B., and P. Shimer. 1990. *Fitness without exercise*. New York: Warner Books.

University of California, Berkeley, School of Public Health. 1991. *The wellness encyclopedia: The comprehensive family resource for safeguarding health and preventing illness*. Boston: Houghton Mifflin.

U.S. Department of Health and Human Services, Public Health Service. 1991. *Healthy people 2000: National health promotion and disease prevention objectives*. DHHS Publication No. (PHS) 91-50212. Washington, DC.

Vickery, D., and J. Fries. 1991. *Take care of yourself: Your personal guide to self-care and preventing illness*. Reading, MA: Addison-Wesley.

Wood, P. 1983. *California diet and exercise program*. Mountain View, CA: Anderson World Books.

Index